Book Descripti

Your heart and mind are constantly racing with anxiety, and you are so desperate you would do anything to put an end to your anxiety and regain control of your brain and body—but what you have tried so far has not worked. You shouldn't beat yourself up, however, because it's not your fault. Your brain has developed, over countless years, the ability to caution you and be ready for fight or flight. The solution you desire is not only a destination, but also a proven process that guides you to a place where you feel peace, have self-control, utilize the life hacks of experts, and be your best self. Your personal path will be very similar to the path from addiction to sobriety: recovery of who you once were before anxiety ensnared you. This quest will free you from what has not helped you in the past and allow you to lead the abundant life you have wished for and deserve in your future.

Anxiety Quest

Guided Adventures: Turning Fear to Courage,
Panic to Calm, Nervous to Confidence

Dr. Ray Wm. Smith

© **Copyright 2022 - All rights reserved.**

The content contained within this book may not be reproduced, duplicated or transmitted without direct written permission from the author or the publisher.

Under no circumstances will any blame or legal responsibility be held against the publisher, or author, for any damages, reparation, or monetary loss due to the information contained within this book, either directly or indirectly.

Legal Notice:

This book is copyright protected. It is only for personal use. You cannot amend, distribute, sell, use, quote or paraphrase any part, or the content within this book, without the consent of the author or publisher.

Disclaimer Notice:

Please note the information contained within this document is for educational and entertainment purposes only. All effort has been executed to present accurate, up to date, reliable, complete information. No warranties of any kind are declared or implied. Readers acknowledge the author is not engaged in the rendering of legal, financial, medical or professional advice. The content within this book has been derived from various sources. Please consult a licensed professional before attempting any techniques outlined in this book.

By reading this document, the reader agrees under no circumstances is the author responsible for any losses, direct or indirect, incurred as a result of the use of the information contained within this document, including, but not limited to, errors, omissions, or inaccuracies.

Table of Contents

Dedication	6
Prologue	7
Introduction: The Quest	9
Chapter 1: Clarifying the Problems with Your Level of Anxiety	13
Types of Anxiety	15
Generalized Anxiety Disorder	16
Obsessive-Compulsive Disorder	16
Panic Disorder	17
Post-Traumatic Stress Disorder	18
Social Anxiety Disorder	19
Performance Anxiety	20
Separation Anxiety Disorder	21
Bottom Line	22
Chapter 2: Starting Your Quest	27
The Science of the Brain	29
The Limbic System	30
Moods	32
Tools for the Mind	33
EFT: Emotional Freedom Technique	36
CBT: Cognitive-Behavioral Therapy	40
Humor	43
The Frequency, Intensity, Duration, and Impact of Your Anxiety	44
Assessments for Anxiety	46
Definitions	48
Courage is Taking a Known Risk For a Known Reward	48
Sobriety	49
Distinctions Between Anxiety and Fear	50
Chapter 3: Developing Courage	55
To Face Your Fears	58
To Feel Your Emotions	60

To End the Impact of Your Past	62
To Forgive Yourself and Everyone Involved	63
To Finally Accept Where...	65
You've Been	66
You Are	66
You Want to Be	67
Chapter 4: Feeling Calm	**71**
Problems With Panic	73
Solutions to Panic Attacks	75
Identifying Triggers	76
Preventing Panic Attacks	78
Tips for Coping	83
Chapter 5: Being Confident	**87**
Problems With Nervousness	89
Performance Anxiety	90
Solutions to Nervousness and Phobias	91
Mindfulness	91
Bodyfulness	92
Pelvic Floor	93
Breathing 4 by 4	93
Fingertip Massage to Yawn	94
Chapter 6: Accepting the Consequences of Failure	**97**
Growth From Failure	99
Alternative Forms of Treatment	100
Medication	100
Hotlines, Helplines, and Online Resources	101
Chapter 7: Celebrating Your Successes	**105**
Recognizing What You Have Achieved	107
Complimenting Yourself	108
Famous People Who Have Overcome Anxiety	108
Conclusion: Helping Others with Anxiety	**113**
Epilogue	**116**

Dedication

Anxiety Quest is dedicated to those who suffer from all forms of anxiety, in the hope of relieving your suffering and help you travel to a place with peace of mind, sobriety, and joy.

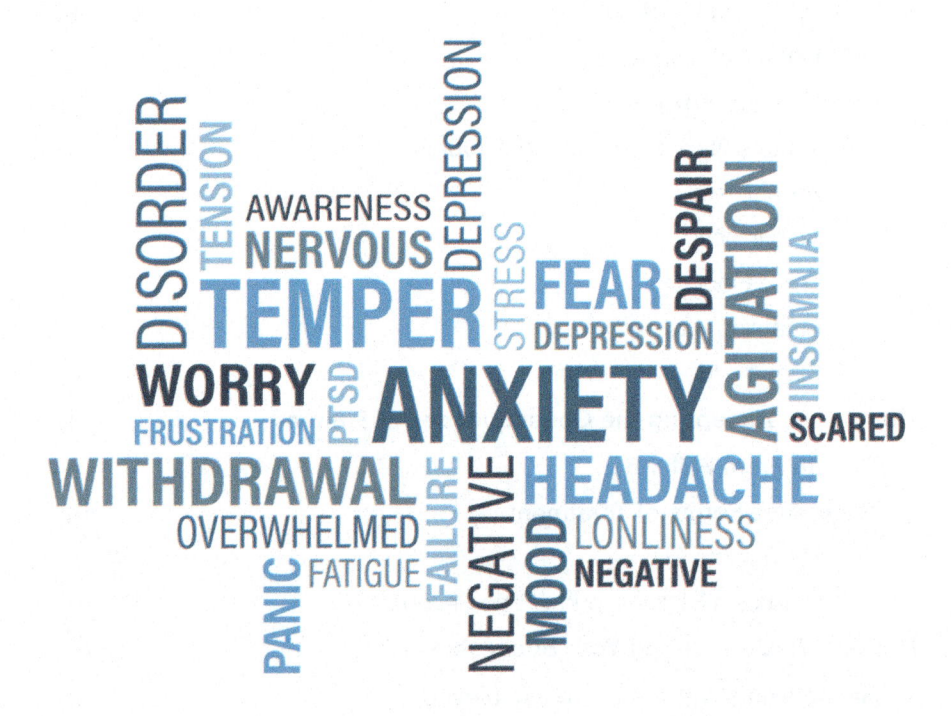

Prologue

> "The reason why it's time to take this quest is because anxiety increased 6 times during COVID"
> - Dr. Ray

If you find you are not satisfied with how often or how long you have felt your anxiety, then you are probably more than ready to begin your journey working toward minimizing your anxiety and promoting your peace of mind. The bad news is overcoming anxiety is not easy. But overcoming it is not without a silver lining; you don't have to find your way completely on your own, and it's more than okay to follow a guide who has achieved, and knows how to direct you to where you want to be. Imagine if you were young King Arthur and had pulled the sword from the stone, only to then need to figure out how to become the best you can be. It would not be easy and would probably foster some worry. To help him with this, King Arthur enlisted the help of Merlin to guide him to become the best version of himself.

Let's get real for a moment: you're not a King and I lack the magic of Merlin. In reality, you have your best self and perhaps can recall times when you felt and behaved at your best. "Okay," you might reply, "but that's not where I am right now!" Which is fair enough. But think back to when you were a toddler, learning to walk—you were not good at it when you first tried and fell left, right, forward, and backward. With time and practice, however, you learned to walk without falling. In a similar vein, with time and practice, you can also learn to master anxiety.

When my children and grandchildren were learning to walk, I walked backward just ahead of them, letting them wrap their little hands around my outstretched fingers, spoke encouragement, while preventing falls, and celebrated with them each step.

I already knew how to walk and had taught others to walk. And I already know how to cope with anxiety and have taught others to walk away from it. I will be honored to guide you too.

Anxiety is the most common mental health problem in America. During the COVID pandemic alone, anxiety became six times more common in the American population and therefore more destructive than ever before. Plagued with worry, our nation, and its citizens are divided about masks, shots, toilet paper shortages, and getting sick or making someone else sick.

This book is not to heal the nation or all its citizens, but rather gently guide you on a quest ending with you being where you want to be, regardless of your background, values, and past. Let's get started toward your destination!

Introduction: The Quest

> "Nothing diminishes anxiety faster than action."
> – Walter Anderson

Sights, sounds, smells, feelings, and flavors—every stimulus you encounter in your human experience is what helps to shape your ideas about the world and your place within it. Both novel and complex, the human experience can be vastly different from one person to the next. For example, a smell someone may associate with good memories and comfort, another may associate with negative thoughts and memories.

Sometimes, but not very frequently, the root of a like or dislike may be easily identified and therefore easily understood. However, in the instance where you may be unable to properly attribute a like or dislike to a solid reason or cause, it can be very frustrating. This especially can be the case when you are being forced to endure highly negative sensations as the result of an un-pinpointed dislike. For most of us, the typical response to these unpleasant feelings is anxiety and its symptoms.

Quite possibly the hardest part of experiencing anxiety is it's largely an automatic bodily response; one in which you don't have much control. The fact this is an automatic response is not necessarily a bad thing, as human brains are hardwired to feel anxious, but it can at times feel excessive, overwhelming, or even debilitating. This doesn't mean tackling and overcoming your anxiety is an impossible task, rather just one needing a committed, multi-step approach with lots of dedication.

There is a distinction to be made, however, specifically between you and every other person who experiences anxiety.

While you and others who are afflicted with anxiety will very likely have a strong desire to be rid of this negative sensation, it is only the individuals like you who are ready to begin their journey. This is because, through just reading this book, you have taken the vital first step in your quest of defeating anxiety. The time is now for you, young padawan, to become the Jedi master and hero you are destined to be!

Take it from me, I understand how hard it can be to walk away from anxiety. You are a brilliant, complex, and novel person who deserves to lead a fulfilling life free of anxious thoughts. Through this book, it is my ultimate goal to guide you successfully on the prosperous quest of learning about, understanding, and finally attaining your sobriety from anxiety.

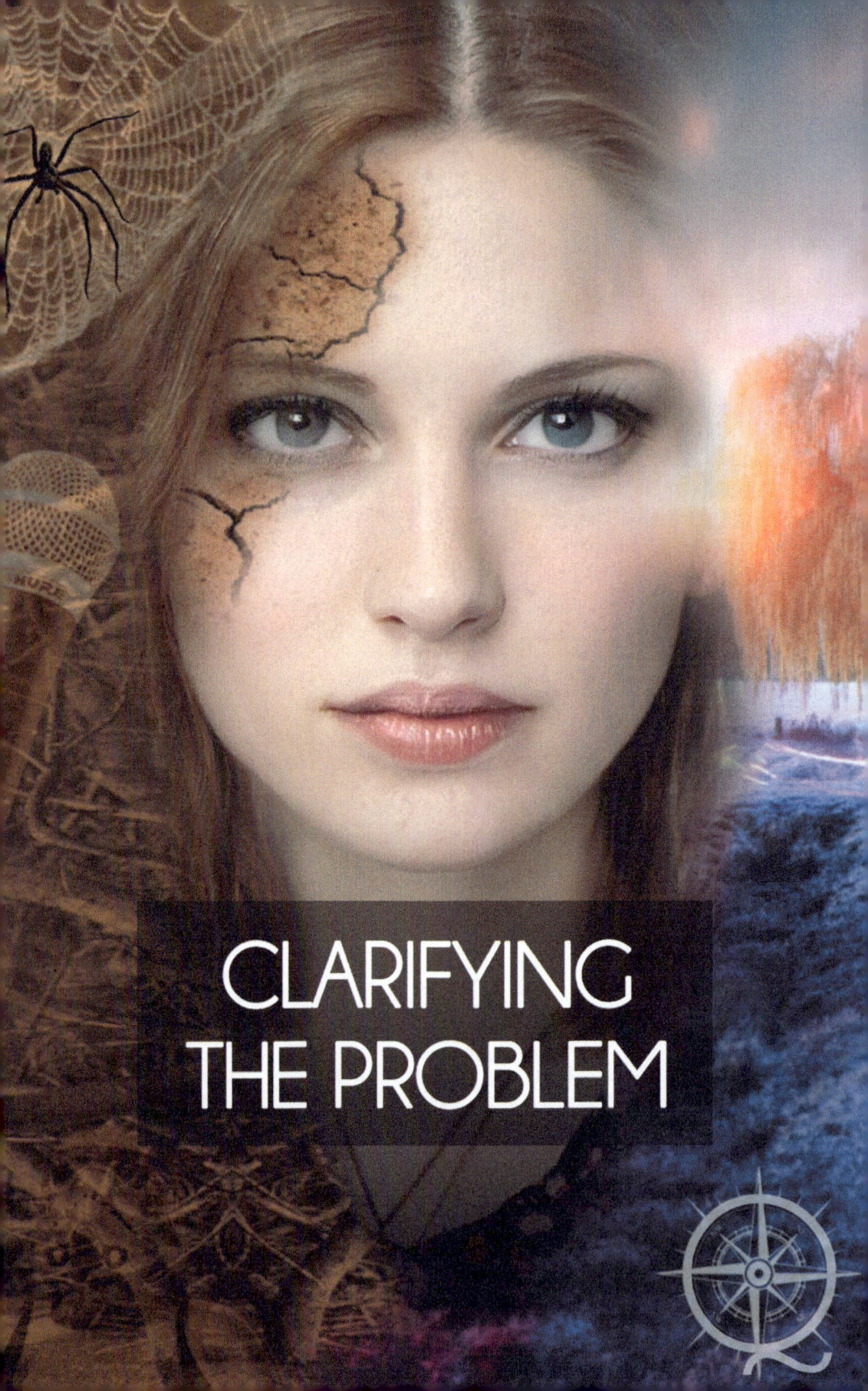

CLARIFYING THE PROBLEM

Chapter 1: Clarifying the Problems with Your Level of Anxiety

As you are probably already aware, anxiety can manifest in us many different ways, through a wide array of factors like genetics, upbringing, and environmental circumstances. Symptoms and feelings of anxiety are typically a sensory response to a very personal set of dimensions. The good news is, while the reasons everyone experiences anxiety can vary from person to person, the general treatment options crafted by psychologists and other mental health professionals, can be applied to all kinds of anxiety and its symptoms.

In order to begin treatment, however, it is best to take the time to develop an awareness of how to classify your anxiety. One of the best ways to solve an issue in a step-by-step manner is to compartmentalize the problem. This is otherwise known as clarifying the problems you have. Whenyou choose to take the time to clarify the details of a problem you are facing, it makes it much easier to envision exactly what you are looking to accomplish by the end of your journey.

Now, I recognize this may be very hard for you to do. I know it is not easy to force yourself to reflect on the symptoms and feelings you experience while feeling anxious, as this means potentially having to relive unsavory experiences and emotions. In the hopes of minimizing this difficult aspectof the process for you, the rest of this chapter will be dedicated to sharing the many different waysanxiety can take form, as well as the surrounding symptoms that typically accompany each kind. By acquiring this knowledge, not only will you then be adequately

"Your mind will answer most questions if you learn to relax and wait for the answer." – William S. Burroughs primed to officially begin your quest, but you may also gain some insight into what you are experiencing, which can help you feel more confident in taking your first step!

Types of Anxiety

In its essence, anxiety is a very robust disorder. Since the majority of an anxious response can be characterized as "autonomic" or "fight or flight", which are terms to be explained in a later chapter, it is far more effective to closely examine the peripheral aspects and details of each kind of anxiety. In doing so, more distinct classes or types of anxiety can be formulated and therefore uniquely catered to in the treatment process. However, for the sake of time and your attention span, the explanations of the different kinds of anxiety will be heavily summarized and not very technically detailed. If you would prefer a complete and more comprehensive list of symptoms for each disorder, please refer to your audiobook companion PDF, which comes free with your purchase, to learn more about these disorders in greater detail.

In addition to this, it is worth mentioning while all of these disorders are different from one another, they all share two criteria in common: first, the symptoms, feelings, and avoidance in which you experience, impair important areas of functioning in your life to a debilitating or clinical degree, and second, the manifestations you experience cannot be explained or attributed to another disorder, medical condition, or physiological effect of a substance.

Generalized Anxiety Disorder

To kick this section off, we will begin by examining Generalized Anxiety Disorder, which is sometimes referred to as GAD. This disorder is distinguished from ordinary anxiety by primarily the intensity and frequency of symptoms experienced by the afflicted person. If you find you experience very severe and frequent manifestations of anxiety, it is likely you could have or could be on the road to having, a case of GAD. Unfortunately, GAD must be treated if identified, as it will only worsen and become more debilitating if neglected. Generalized Anxiety Disorder can also be exhibited through:

- You feel an exaggerated level of anxiety and worry over a wide array of events and circumstances
- This exaggerated anxiety or worry feels impossible to control and weighs you down significantly
- You have been feeling these excessive feelings for at least six months

Obsessive-Compulsive Disorder

One fascinating thing about anxiety, which also happens to be one of the reasons why there are different levels and degrees of this affliction, is it can demonstrate itself in an assortment of ways. Because of this, it can sometimes be quite hard for you to identify your disorder, simply due to how uniquely the disorder is presenting itself. This idea holds true for many different kinds of anxiety but begins to fall short when examining a disorder named Obsessive Compulsive Disorder, which is most commonly known as OCD. OCD is designated as a special type of anxiety, meaning a clinical diagnosis is only officially provided for you if you meet all of the unique criteria most recently established and agreed upon by the international psychological community. Usually, OCD is identified by the presence of either obsessions, compulsions, or both. In a bit more detail, the criteria of OCD can be summarized by the following:

- You feel excessive levels of anxiety as a result of experiencing intrusive and unwanted obsessions, which take the form of incessant thoughts, images, or urges
- These obsessions are unavoidable, no matter how hard you try
- You must engage in and feel tied to hyper-specific, repetitive behaviors or cognitions known as compulsions, and failure to engage in those compulsions brings you extreme distress or discomfort
- These obsessions or compulsions affect you for at least one hour per day

Panic Disorder

Since you now have a basic understanding of GAD, it is important to learn about a disorder principally believed to be intertwined within it, Panic Disorder. Like GAD, panic disorder develops when left untreated. The big difference is, that while generalized anxiety disorder stems simply from untreated anxiety, panic disorder stems from untreated GAD.

This means if you are afflicted with GAD and try to avoid or put off treatment, you would be running the risk of your initial disorder developing into a different, more acute one. PD can take the form of just usual panic attacks, where you may or may not know the triggers, or as agoraphobia, where specific public situations are triggering you. To be diagnosed with panic disorder you must also experience:

- You often are faced with either expected or unexpected panic attacks and feel relentless concern over future panic attacks and their consequences
- If you know your triggers, you actively avoid situations where you may cross paths with them at all costs
- The level of panic you experience is grossly disproportionate to the circumstance triggering it and has happened at least once per month

Post-Traumatic Stress Disorder

Post-Traumatic Stress Disorder, otherwise known as PTSD, is probably the most complex out of all the kinds of anxiety shared in this section. Unlike GAD, OCD, and PD, which are all suspected to have at least some form of genetic predisposition tied to their presence, PTSD is developed entirelydue to your experiences with your outside environment. Since there is a long list of criteria to be met to satisfy the clinical standard of this affliction, PTSD can be taken as a one-of-a-kind type of anxiety diagnosed as all or nothing. When severe, PTSD can be the most debilitating form of anxiety and can completely change a person from who they once were. In short, PTSD is marked by the presence of:

- You have been exposed to an intensely horrifying, threatening, or gruesome event by way of proxy or personal experience
- You experience several intrusive symptoms regularly you find very distressing and are related to the memory of the disturbing event
- Any sort of interaction with any aspect of this memory results in marked, negative changes to your mood, awareness, responses, or treatment of others
- You maintain a steadfast avoidance of anything related to the traumatic memory

Social Anxiety Disorder

Compared to the other kinds of anxiety listed in this section, Social Anxiety Disorder is likely to be the type you are most familiar with. This is largely because almost every person in their lifetime has experienced some form of social anxiety at one time or another. However, experiencing social anxiety from time to time is a far more toned-down version of social anxiety disorder, which is clinical. Those who are faced with this affliction typically experience crippling levels of anxiety in response to even the idea of being in a social situation. A disorder of this kind can act as asignificant hindrance to a person's ability to develop basic socialization skills and prevent them from ever being fully integrated into society. For example, some of my patients refused to go inside a big box store. If you were afflicted with social anxiety disorder you would experience:

- Feeling a protracted sense of anxiety and or fear in response to, or even the idea of, certain social situations where you could be privy to criticism, for at least six months
- You avoid these identified social situations to the fullest degree, otherwise to be endured with unmanageable distress
- Your anxious and or fearful response is highly unequal to the actual threat level presented

Performance Anxiety

Performance Anxiety, while not officially a clinical disorder, is usually viewed as a facet of social anxiety. As it is almost identical in symptoms and criteria to social anxiety, the only distinction between the two is people with performance anxiety will primarily experience their symptoms when being observed or having to present publicly in front of others. Unfortunately, the exact prevalence rates of performance anxiety are not known and often get grouped in with the overall prevalence rate of social anxiety disorder. The one thing that can be said for certain, however, is markers of performance anxiety have been reported within the population of pretty much every developed country in the world. I am writing this during the Winter Olympics in China, where every athlete feels some level of performance anxiety.

Seeing it would be quite redundant to relist the criteria and symptoms of social anxiety disorder again, which is the framework used to diagnose performance anxiety as well, please refer back to the section on social anxiety disorder when looking to examine the criteria necessary for performance anxiety. In light of recent events, I feel as though it is worthwhile to mention public speaking generates enough social anxiety that surveys across America found a sizable percentage of the population are more afraid of talking before a group than they are of COVID, cancer, or car collisions. As a student in school, if you ever had dry mouth and found yourself worried about making a mistake or looking foolish, then you may dread giving a talk even now. In fact, many athletes, comedians, and actors have anxiety about their upcoming performance, sometimes so severe they don't perform and feel a lowered self-esteem.

Separation Anxiety Disorder

On the surface, it may seem as though experiencing a bit of separation anxiety is not a bad thing. Intruth, separation anxiety can be a good thing. It is a fabulous marker of someone building relationships and making connections with other people, places, and things around us. To a limited degree, separation helps us be social creatures who look to one another in a time of need. But like all good things, separation can be taken too far and become excessive. When this happens, it usually means that the person is afflicted with it. Separation anxiety can be very tricky—it can be hard to bring yourself to medicalize an attachment you have to someone or something. However, this kind of disorder mustn't carry on unaddressed, as separation anxiety not only deeply affects the person experiencing it, but also the figures of attachment who are subject to the person's treatment. While some separation may be justified, when it is to a degree of being an imposition for any party involved, it must be treated. Separation anxiety disorder is characterized by:

- You experience an uncontrollable level of anxiety, fear, or distress in response to separation, whether legitimate or imagined, from your figure of attachment
- You do everything in your power to prevent or minimize separation from your figure of attachment
- Your feelings surrounding separation and outright avoidance of it have persisted for at least six months

Bottom Line

Ultimately, when taking the time to examine anxiety as a whole on a more abstract level, it can viably be boiled down to your response of fear, experiencing a traumatic event, feeling inadequate, or being rejected. Understanding this fact is vital to your ability to start your quest off on the right foot and to know what is to come on the road ahead. Whether you are someone who is afflicted with a clinical disorder or struggles with anxiety here and there, having rich knowledge and a tight grasp of what anxiety is, and how you personally experience it, is all you need to take your first step on this rewarding journey.

> "Find a Guide who knows your state of mind and where you want to be."—Dr. Ray

I am an Eagle Scout. The only way to become an Eagle Scout is for the older boys to help you achieve your goals along the same path they traveled. They guide a Scout from Tenderfoot through all the ranks and Merit Badges needed to **Be Prepared**, the primary purpose of the journey toward leadership. Perhaps it makes sense now to follow the trail of a leader who knows where you want to go, why the trip is worth it to you and can take you there because they've been there ahead of you.

Allow this book to serve you as Merlin for the young King Arthur. Let's take the first step together.

LEFT OPEN FOR NOTES

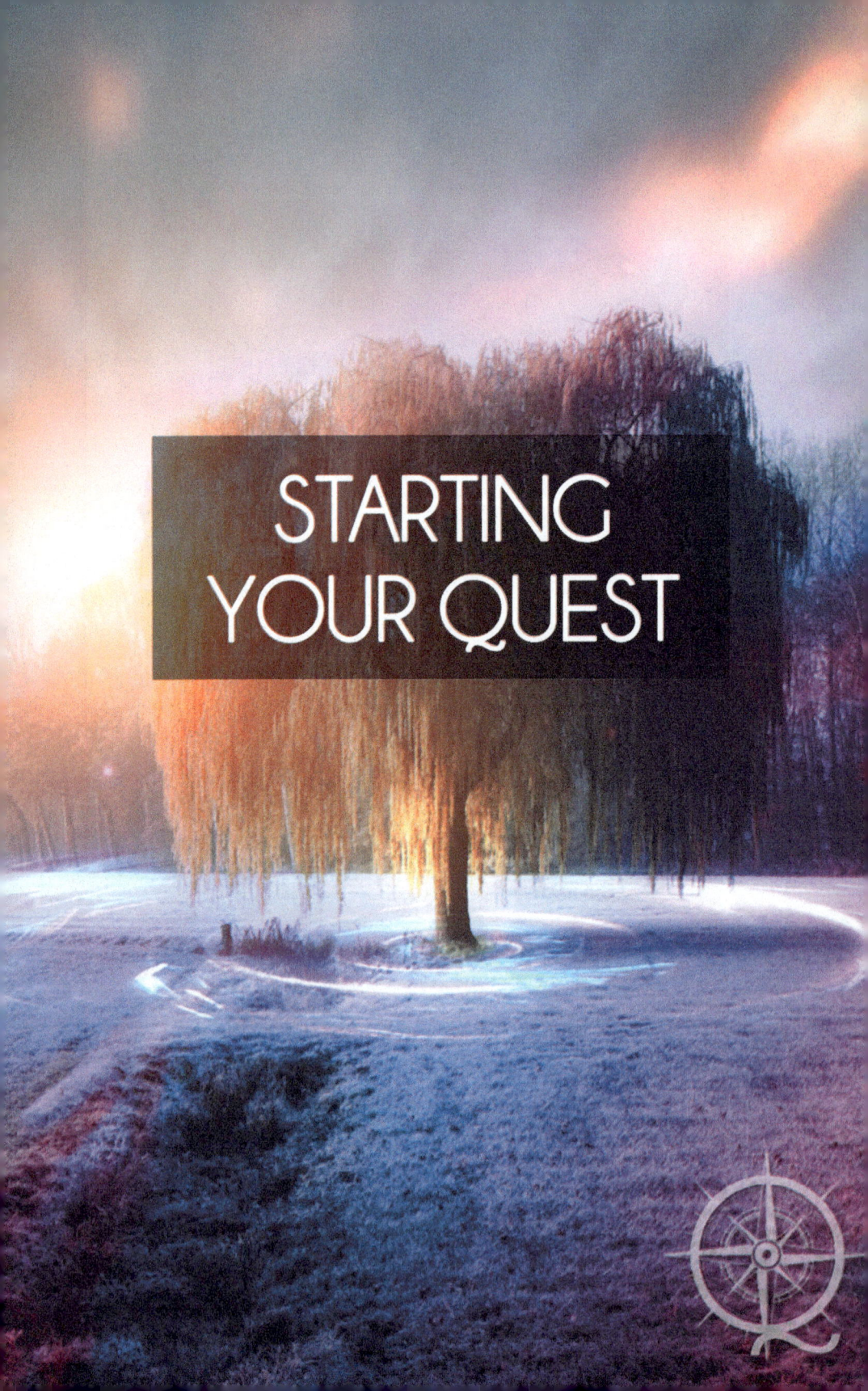

STARTING YOUR QUEST

Chapter 2: Starting Your Quest

Before getting into the details, I feel as though the best way to begin this chapter would be to share a short anecdote about my son and his struggle with anxiety.

Growing up, one of my sons had a phobia of spiders. As the weather got colder in Spokane Washington, the spiders found their way into our home, his room, and the hallway next to the garage. Any time he came across a spider, he would shriek at the sight of it. However, because I felt compassion for his anxiety, I would take the time to remove any, if not all, of the spiders I would come across. If he was left home alone with them, he would squash them as fast as he could, leaving the residue on the floor or walls. He would leave their unfortunate bodies where they had died, in the hopes the other spiders would learn from it and seek refuge somewhere else.

As expected, to my son's dismay, the spiders stayed. However, although the spiders clearly had no intention of leaving, my son gradually learned to defeat his fear and find his power. Through this, he managed to develop the confidence necessary to know how to react appropriately when faced with future spiders.

My son's story of how he overcame his phobia of spiders is a perfect example of the personal journey to be taken when looking to rid yourself of anxiety. Every person's quest is unique and should be closely catered to meet their wants and needs, seeing we live in a unique, diverse world with all kinds of individuals. When embarking upon a personal quest such as

"You can't always control what goes on outside. But you can always control what goes on inside." –Wayne Dyer this one, the only finish line you should be looking towards is the one you, and you alone, have set for yourself. While there are noissues with receiving help or guidance on this quest, you will be far better served with the knowledge and awareness of all the resources at your disposal enabling you to progress forward.

Since you now have a solid base of knowledge and understanding of many different types of anxiety and their officially recognized symptoms, the next best step is to take the time to learn and develop an understanding of the science behind the part of the brain allowing you to feel these anxious symptoms, as well as the tools and assessments you have to choose from while pursuing your journey.

The Science of the Brain

Before jumping in, it is worth noting the details shared in this section, while helpful, are rather technical in nature and can be a bit confusing at times. If you find the details of this section to be too complex, or simply don't have much interest in learning about the different parts of the brain, it is completely okay to fast forward to the other practical tools shared in this chapter to be utilized regardless of your background and understanding. On the other hand, if you want to learn more about all the technical details of the limbic system, please refer to your free audiobook companion PDF.

The human brain is truthfully a marvelous but mysterious organ—it controls every area of ourfunctioning and acts largely as the communication headquarters within our bodies, yet we know so little about how it really works in the grand scheme of things. One of the things we know for sure, however, is you are your brain. This means when something is out of balance with us emotionally or mentally, the problem resides directly within our brains rather than anywhere else in our bodies.

Building off this, it seems only logical to properly and adequately address an issue going on within our brains, we should try to gain as much of an understanding as we can, from many different dimensions. Included in this, is learning about the specific systems in the brain, how they are organized, and how they can affect us mentally or emotionally, especially in the case of feeling off or unbalanced. In the case of anxiety, there are many different brain mechanisms and subsystems involved in making us feel the way we do when we feel anxious. One system in particular that stands out in this process, however, is the exceptionally important limbic system. The limbic system serves many purposes in the human brain but is generally most responsible for emotional and behavioral responses to various stimuli.

The Limbic System

Just by developing a basic understanding of it, it is more than obvious just how intricate dissecting the human brain can be.

The limbic system makes up just one of the numerous systems operating in your brain that makes you the person you are. In addition to the roles it plays on its own, the limbic system is also involved in a much larger, grand scale processes in your brain affecting your entire body. An example of this is how the limbic system plays a key role in activating your body's automatic response when it senses danger. This is known as activating your autonomic nervous system or rather as your fight-or-flight response. Your autonomic nervous system executes several different functions to prepare your body to respond adequately in a time of intense distress. How your limbic system works to play a role in this bodily response is by helping to identify the stimulus of the perceived threat.

In addition to helping to activate your fight-or-flight response, your limbic system plays a role in your learning, emotional and behavioral responses, storing knowledge, and the formation and retention of new memories. As you can probably guess, this system has many different components to it, with each component playing a necessary part in the system's function. The six structures making up the limbic system are: the **Hippocampus**, the **Amygdala**, the **Cingulate Gyrus**, the **Thalamus**, the **Hypothalamus**, and the **Basal Ganglia**. Should damage ever occur to any of these structures, it is likely you would be rendered unable to ever make proper use of your limbic system again. While not physical in nature, the damage excessive anxiety can cause and how it interacts with the limbic system is quite intriguing and novel.

To provide some context on these substructures, the rest of this section will focus on the general important details of how each one specifically interacts with anxiety.

The **Hippocampus** is the structure responsible for the formation and consolidation of memory. It is believed this is also where your anxiety triggers and distressing anxiety-related memories are stored, which primes your brain to be sensitive to specific circumstances.

Another structure nearby is the **Amygdala**, which is responsible for emotions and emotion-laden behavioral responses. If you experience chronic anxiety, your **Amygdala** is far more likely to be much more sensitive than the average person, as anxiety causes it to remain on high alert for potential triggers. This can lead to further out of whack emotional responses if anxiety goes without being treated.

Without getting too complicated, the **Basal Ganglia** is a substructure made up of more substructures. In sum, the **Basal Ganglia** works to help with habit formation, and primes your brain for more anxious responses if you have had one or several in the past.

The **Thalamus** and **Hypothalamus**, both similar in name, are very different in terms of importance and function. While the **Thalamus** operates in the regulation of motor responses and sensory perception, the **Hypothalamus** orchestrates a lot of different functions since it's involved in many automatic bodily processes such as thirst, body temperature, and heart rate.

The **Hypothalamus** also works to release and mediate hormones as well as integrate stimuli. The fact it is an integration center is what allows for it to be very affected by unmediated anxiety—the more regular the stress, the more likely it is to misinterpret the stimuli.

In all of this, the **Cingulate Gyrus** functions as the pathway connecting incoming stimuli to the rest of the limbic system, so any sort of damage can lead to developing the inability to elicit a fearful response altogether.

Moods

Not only is the limbic system responsible for almost all emotional and behavioral responses, but it also largely controls and mediates our moods. The specific system of interest to moods in the Limbic system is the **Amygdala**. Responsible not only for detecting stimuli and provoking emotions, but works very closely with the moods we experience. Any damage the **Amygdala** faces acts as a serious threat to our ability to regulate our moods, emotions, and to respond appropriately when necessary.

As a result, someone with a damaged **Amygdala** could be more likely to put themselves in harm's way because they are unable to properly feel fear, or could be more likely to exhibit a disproportionate aggressive response to a nonaggressive stimulus. Damage to the **Amygdala**, while not very common, is a factor to be considered when determining the path in which you would like to follow on your quest to sobriety from anxiety, as this can alter how you should approach it. If you suspect that your **Amygdala** or any part of your limbic system really has damage, it is best to reach out to a professional who is qualified to confirm whether this is the case or not, as soon as you can.

Tools for the Mind

When examining fictional stories of individuals with great heroism, such as King Arthur of Camelot or the Jedi knights of Star Wars, there are several shared aspects about each story typically falling under the literary trope of a hero's journey to success. Wit, strength, courage, and charm— the heroes of these kinds of stories tend to possess it all. An important caveat to consider while reveling in these positive qualities these heroes ascribe dutifully to, is none of these heroes became heroes overnight. In Star Wars, Jedi training for young Padawans begins at a young age, and the stories of King

Arthur begin chronicling from the time he is fifteen and continue well into his adulthood. Each and every one of these heroes had a journey in which they committed to and followed, developing their desirable qualities of heroism along the way. While these stories may be fictional, this concept can without a doubt also be applied to the very real quest you are looking to take yourself on.

The idea behind this is your quest will take time, and similar to the heroes in Arthurian legends and Star Wars, your best chance of success is to not try to do it alone. Now, this does not necessarilymean your success is entirely dependent on how often you look to others for help during your quest, but rather it depends on your ability to be open to all kinds of tools and resources available to you. After all, King Arthur and the Jedi didn't just source their power purely from within, but also through the alliances they formed on their quest as well as the weapons they use in battle.

Your mind is an amazing thing, capable of more than you think —but it can be extremely difficult to harness this power without having the proper tools to do so. These tools can vary widely, depending on the person. For King Arthur, his tools were the sword, Excalibur, and the wizard Merlin, which is quite different from the tools of the Jedi, who used the force and lightsabers.

Ultimately, your quest will consist of applying your unique set of mind tools that you have chosen to help you along the way. On top of this, your personal set of mind tools are highly flexible and can be altered or swapped out in any way that best suits you, because mindfulness is a commonly used tool to master anxiety. While a recent study reported sometimes, for some people, mindfulness can actually produce more anxiety, I do not believe this fact should ever deter anyone from trying out mindfulness. Like the old commercials say, "Try it. You'll like it!". You may like one tool and maybe not, but the only way to learn is through trial and error.

At this point, as I write this, I feel as though it is worth mentioning I have a patient who has been using cannabis as an anti-anxiety medication, even though it is an illegal substance at the teen's age. As so often happens, the use and abuse of weed was discovered when the A student's grades literally went to pot! Willie Nelson might say marijuana is best for him, but it was not best for my patient, as their misguided trial and error came at the expense of their own college and career goals.

The best place to start when deciding which mind tools you would like to try, however, is by learningabout all the different kinds of tools and resources, which range anywhere from formal therapy to finding a new hobby available to you when planning your journey. Through gaining this knowledge, you will have a much clearer idea of which methods you believe work best, and which ones you should avoid. Never forget, this quest is deeply personal and the process cannot be rushed in order to make certain in the methods you have chosen to apply will work. You will find through taking your time during this step, success will come far more easily—all just because you have taken the time to be certain about what works best for you.

For example, if you had a physical medical problem, you would probably opt to begin addressing it by educating yourself about the treatment options available. Usually, the initial treatment options most heavily considered are the ones least harmful and yield the least amount of side effects. So by applying this logic, if your doctor gave you a diagnosis and advised you amputation would be best, you might seek a second opinion suggesting an alternative form of treatment with a minimal impact, in order to save the radical surgery for last, if the other options fail.

EFT: Emotional Freedom Technique

The Emotional Freedom Technique, also known as EFT, is a simple yet effective treatment method engaging you both physically and mentally. Targeted to relieve physical discomfort and emotional distress, this technique is primarily tapping your body a series of times to treat physical discomfort or pain and foster a balance of your internal energy. This technique has been coined by Gary Craig, who views disrupted energy as the cause of all negative feelings, emotions, discomfort, and pain.

Personally, I am a strong supporter of EFT because it has the ability to change your brain through a series of electricity currents by way of your nerves, as well as change your mindset by programming yourself to engage in healthier cognitions, or ways of thinking about anxiety. To help you with understanding this technique, I suggest an internet search of videos teaching you how to use EFT for anxiety. You will find there are a variety of ways to use EFT to help annihilate anxiety, and there have never been any reported negative side effects of giving it a try. You really might like it!

If you are unfamiliar with the emotional freedom technique, you are probably wondering how exactly a series of taps on your body produces such a strong effect. Well, EFT is somewhat like acupuncture; you are looking to target very specific points of your body, otherwise known as energy hot spots or meridian points. The concept of meridian points on the human body is based on the knowledge of Chinese herbal medicine, which believes these points on your body are where energy flows.

These energy hot spots are what balance your energy and therefore maintain your health. Whenever your energy is unbalanced, you are left vulnerable to illness and negative experiences. The purpose of the tapping is to replace the acupuncture needles typically used to access these points and to send signals to the area of your brain responsible for stress. Through this, it is believed you are able to reduce the negative disruptions and restore your energy once again. Results from this technique can easily be attained just by applying these five steps.

The first step of the emotional freedom technique is to identify the issue you are looking to target and eliminate. This is important to the effectiveness of the technique, primarily because this will dictate where the focal point of your tapping will be directed. To truly reap the benefits of this technique, it is highly recommended you focus solely on one issue at a time, as doing so is believed to enhance the end results in positive ways.

Once the dimensions of your issue have been established, the next step is to determine the intensity of the discomfort you are feeling. The intensity scale used for this technique is from zero to ten, with ten being the highest intensity of the discomfort. By determining the intensity of your discomfort, you are able to be more cognizant of how your feelings of discomfort change as you continue with the exercise. In addition to this, determining the intensity of your discomfort teaches and promotes staying in tune with your emotions and feelings, which is a fundamental component of anxiety sobriety.

The last step before you can begin your tapping ritual is to try your hardest to verbalize the issue you are seeking to address in a short phrase. The only criteria to be met for this phrase is to acknowledge the issue and accept yourself despite the problem. An example of a phrase structure you could use is, "Although I am faced with this issue, I sincerely and wholly accept myself." This phrase can be tweaked in any way that best suits you, as long as it is not addressing the issue of someone else. The idea behind this is you must be able to pinpoint and dial in on how the issue makes you feel in order to relieve yourself from the distress it is causing you.

Next, is to finally begin the tapping step of this technique. The emotional freedom technique tapping sequence is a systematic pattern of taps upon nine of your meridian points. There are twelve meridian points mirroring each other on your body in total, with each point corresponding with a different organ in your body. However, the nine points the emotional freedom technique focuses on are:

1. The karate chop, which corresponds with the small intestine meridian
2. The top of the head, which is a governing energy vessel
3. The eyebrow, which corresponds with the bladder meridian
4. The side of the eye, which corresponds with the gallbladder meridian
5. Under the eye, which corresponds with the stomach meridian
6. Under the nose, which is a governing energy vessel
7. The chin, which is a central energy vessel
8. The beginning of the collarbone, which corresponds with the kidney meridian
9. Under the arm, which corresponds with the spleen meridian

This sequence is begun by starting with tapping the karate chop point, which is the side of your hand opposite from your thumb, while simultaneously repeating your setup phrase three times in a row. Start with tapping with the fingerprint edge of each finger on your opposite hand, between the end of the wrist and the start of your pinkie finger. Next, tap each of the following points seven times, beginning at the top, descending down your body:

- Your eyebrow
- The side of your eye
- Under your eye

- Under your nose
- Your chin
- The beginning of your collar bone
- Under your arm

Once you have finished tapping under your arm, the sequence is completed by ending at the top of your head. While you tap throughout your body, think of a small reminder phrase you can say to yourself. Be sure to say this phrase at each tapping point at least once. Ideally, what you say the firsttime is the truth of the negative aspects of your anxiety. This can sound something like: "I hate being so nervous and feeling inadequate because of it", or "I feel like I am not measuring up and everyone will see me as an imposter". This sequence should then be completed an additional few more times, as completing it once is usually not enough to bring relief from negative issues entirely.

The last step of the emotional freedom technique is to once again reevaluate the level of intensity in which you are feeling discomfort from your issue. You can then use this assessment as a comparison to the intensity level you felt, before completing the technique, as a means of determining how effective it is for solving your issues. Because the goal of this technique is to bring you back down to an intensity level of zero, these five steps should be repeated until you feel as though you have reached your baseline once again. There is no shame in having to repeat this multiple times in a row for a single issue, as it is better to take the time and put in the work needed to find genuine relief from whatever is causing the imbalance in your energy. If you need to, take a deep breath, and then complete your tapping sequence again, saying the positive things you want to manifest instead of the negative thoughts you said in the previous round. Some examples of the positive things you can say to yourself are: "I wonder if I could repurpose my nervousness as excitement to excel? What if I am enough for this?", or "I know I can do this if I keep my eyes on the prize", or even "I want to practice enough to make it look easy for all those watching me".

CBT: Cognitive-Behavioral Therapy

Cognitive-Behavioral Therapy, known as CBT, is a form of psychological talk therapy widely used by many psychotherapists internationally in treating patients afflicted with depression and anxiety. CBThas been proven to be highly effective in treating anxiety-based disorders by guiding users on how topermanently alter the specific thought patterns instigating the negative symptoms of their illness. An essential facet of effective CBT treatment is something called psychoeducation, which is the act of learning about psychological issues. It is fundamentally believed amongst practitioners of CBT the very critical first step of treating a psychological issue is to become educated on what it is and how itaffects you.

There are many different focal points in the treatment of CBT, meaning this type of therapy is viewed as more of a multi-faceted approach. Similar to EFT, cognitive-behavioral therapy seeks to balance your energy but uses a bit of a different approach to doing so. Instead of a sequence of taps to focus on an issue, negative thoughts and feelings are isolated and interchanged with more balanced and realistic replacements. By practicing realistic thinking, it becomes easier over time to be more aware of the negative thought patterns causing you to spiral and put a halt to them before they provoke a negative emotional response. The process of challenging negative thoughts in place of positive ones takes time to successfully develop but is highly rewarding once achieved and significantly decreases the chances of relapse.

In addition to practicing realistic thinking, cognitive behavioral therapy also teaches a variety of different relaxation strategies. Relaxation in itself can be a tricky thing to do for some of us, but it is more than necessary to understand how to gain the most from treatment. For people who are afflicted with anxiety, learning about relaxation techniques and how to properly use them can be massively helpful since many of the physical symptoms can be counteracted just through simple physical relaxation concepts. The point of relaxation strategies is not to completely get rid of anxiety, but to alleviate the feelings, at least in part, so they are more manageable when you are in a situation where an anxiety-induced emotional response would be highly inappropriate.

The more time you take and effort you put into building and working on these strategies, the more efficient and effective the strategies will be. If you are interested in further reading on CBT, the leading CBT psychiatrist David Burns has developed a vast array of practical applications geared to overcoming anxiety through his many books and podcasts. In addition, you may also want to consider taking a look at www.feelinggood.com, which is another resource with numerous CBT-based applications for treating anxiety.

On top of this, another aspect of CBT specifically used for those afflicted with anxiety is exposuretherapy. Interestingly, exposure therapy is the method believed to be what makes a true difference intreating anxiety. This is because exposure therapy focuses on putting patients in situations or circumstances where they are forced to face their fears. While the idea of it is terrifying to many, through the practice of exposure therapy, you can become more desensitized to whatever is causing you distress. Eventually, with gradual exposure, you are able to get to a point of having little to no reaction to a stimulus invoking extreme discomfort or distress. This makes exposure therapy a highly effective treatment option, especially for those looking to rid themselves of an irrational fear-producing anxious response, and wants help managing their anxiety for the long term.

One of my patients suffered from a phobia of riding in an elevator, which you can only imagine made life exceedingly difficult. Rationally, elevators are one of the safest forms of transportation. (Ironically, the Otis elevator building in Spokane Washington was only one story tall, which may have reinforced the idea, that people in the know will not ride them.) We began exposure therapy with the uncomfortable talk about elevators, safety, and being out of control. During this process, I shared with them the story of a friend who was trapped for several hours in a hot, humid elevator in Thailand, where safety standards are far less than in the US. My friend chose to think someone would come to fix the elevator and decided to lie down and go to sleep until the door opened.

The story, of course, made the patient even more uncomfortable. I pointed out the only option available was to think about getting rescued, relax, and wait patiently while napping. Taking this into consideration, my patient then decided if my 80-year-old friend could overcome anxiety over there, his phobia could be overcome in any elevator. In the session following this realization, we looked at photographs and videos of elevators, and the safety mechanisms they have today. The next session we went to a building nearby and just looked at the elevator coming and going with passengers entering and exiting without a care. Over the next few sessions, the exposure broadened as we eventually began doing an exercise where we stepped in and stepped out of the elevator, then did some progressive relaxation. The final time we went, we rode up one floor and back down, then to the top and back down. The only negative outcome at the end of our work together was the patient feeling silly for ever feeling anxious, which we disputed and refuted with rational cognitions.

Humor

Sometimes when the going gets tough with life, solace can be easily found through the use of humor. As you probably so often hear, laughter is the best medicine, so maintaining a sense of humor can act as a protective factor against developing and worsening mental illness.

However, it is important to note the kind of humor you are engaging in, matters significantly in terms of the mediating effect it can have on your mental health. According to a study completed in the year 2020 on the role of humor in mental illness severity, the kind of humor we partake in can be highly predictive of the state of our mental wellbeing (Menéndez-Aller et al., 2020).

Many years ago, when author Norman Cousins was afflicted with a deadly disease, he decided he wanted to die laughing. He watched old comedies all day long until a friend asked how much time Norman had left. He returned to the doctor, had many tests, and was released with no sign of his medical problems. If he could use mind over matter for physical health, perhaps you could use your sense of humor to feel less anxious.

More specifically, the researchers found those who engage in positive types of humor, such as situational humor, were far less likely to be afflicted with depression or anxiety. In a similar vein, they also found people who engaged in negative types of humor, such as self-deprecating humor, were much more likely to be afflicted with depression or anxiety. The results yielded by this study suggest the kind of humor you practice and ascribe to could either be helping or hindering the effects of your anxiety. So while it may not be humor alone dictating the state of your mental wellbeing, it is never a bad idea to start becoming more conscious of your style of humor and how it could be throwing you off course from your ultimate goal of being anxiety-free.

In the past, Reader's Digest magazine had a column each month called "Laughter Is The Best Medicine", which shared clean jokes. Since then, many comics have told jokes which are way more vulgar and far less helpful in boosting your mood. Personally, I prefer humor that seeks to build up the listener. Recently, I saw Rita Rudner's live show and thought I would have to leave before it ended because my abdomen hurt from laughing so hard for so long. After her performance, I felt great. Sometimes, humor can really be the best medicine.

The Frequency, Intensity, Duration, and Impact of Your Anxiety

When looking to understand your anxiety, the use of introspection can be key to developing an accurate analysis. As stated before, understanding your mental affliction is absolutely imperative to ridding yourself of it. This includes being able to accurately identify the frequency, intensity, duration, and impact of the markers and manifestations you experience. By taking the time to do so, you are doing yourself a massive favor, by isolating the exact problem areas to be addressed in order to promote your sobriety. For example, you may realize only after some self-reflection that the worst aspect of your anxiety is actually the intensity of it rather than the frequency, which is what you previously assumed.

Through analyzing a variety of different dimensions, you can more readily focus on how you can take steps to minimize the level of each dimension, one at a time. If you were to attempt to try andminimize the severity of all of these dimensions at once, you are not only setting yourself up to become quickly overwhelmed but are also significantly less likely to adequately give each dimension the time and focus required to make irreversible positive changes to the state of your affliction.

Outside of introspection, there are many ways you can assess your anxious feelings; both professionally and personally. There is a great degree of flexibility in the kinds of assessments you can choose from, but it is best to exercise caution in bending the rules of practice, as straying too far away from the established framework of an assessment can yield inaccurate results.

Often, many people who are looking to treat their anxiety find the already existing structure of most assessment methods work quite well with little to no alterations, so this is unlikely to be a very significant point of concern on your quest. On top of this, assigning a number to your feelings can be a very easy thing to do, especially when techniques like EFT require you to evaluate your current level of nervousness on a numbered scale. I tend to like to use a method of this sort for children, as it provides them with a simple way to express how they feel and find their gauge just through the act of raising my hand low, middle, or high. By doing this, I can allow them to decide which level best represents how they feel.

Assessments for Anxiety

The information shared in this section on assessments is largely summarized for the sake of brevity. If you are interested in learning more about these assessments in greater detail, please refer to Appendix C in your audio-book companion PDF.

As more and more research studies on anxiety are conducted, more and more assessments are created and used to assess them. As you already know, anxiety is an illness manifesting in a series of unique disorders with distinct characteristics from one to the next. Anxiety assessments are quite accessible and can both be clinician and individually administered.

If you are someone who experiences anxiety and suspect you may be suffering from a disorder, a good place to start is with general anxiety assessments to confirm whether what you are feeling is actually anxiety or can be attributed to some other factor. This can also be helpful in the circumstance where your scores are within the normal range and can reinforce your desire to seek professional help. Some examples of general anxiety assessments are the Beck Anxiety Inventory and the Hamilton Anxiety Rating Scale.

If you suspected you were experiencing symptoms of generalized anxiety disorder, the good news is there is a wide array of assessments from which you can choose. However, two assessments you could look into are the Generalized Anxiety Scale and the Generalized Anxiety Disorder Severity Scale.

For Obsessive Compulsive Disorder on the other hand, unfortunately, there are not very many tests that exist, as there is only one test recently created and is still viewed as the gold standard in terms of OCD assessment. Currently, the most pervasive assessment for OCD available is the Yale-Brown Obsessive-Compulsive Scale. Due to the limited amount of assessments, testing for OCD can only be administered via a clinician.

While it may be a bit counterintuitive due to its lack of generality much like OCD, PTSD has more than a handful of regularly used assessments. These vary greatly, but there exist far more clinician-administered assessments than personally administered ones. Each assessment seeks to target slightly different symptoms the person could be experiencing to define the dimensions of their case. One of the most popular self-administered assessments for PTSD is the Davidson Trauma Scale. Aside from this, some clinician-administered assessments include: the Clinician Administered PTSD scale or DSM-5 and the PTSD Symptom Scale Interview.

Despite how common this next kind of disorder is, there are only a few assessments to test for Social Anxiety Disorder. The majority of these assessments are self-report and are widely accessible including the Liebowitz Social Anxiety Scale and the Social Phobia Inventory.

Unfortunately, due to how newly recognized Separation Anxiety Disorder is, there is no official assessment widely used across this discipline yet, and much more research is required before an adequate one may be created. When looking to assess specific phobias, there are three decidedly popular self-administered assessments usually favored. An important caveat about these specific phobia assessments is, that it is highly recommended the results are followed up by a clinician, as self-assessment is not enough on its own. These self-administered assessments are the Phobia Questionnaire, the Fear Questionnaire, and the Specific Phobia Questionnaire.

Definitions

Before ending this chapter, it would be best to get a few remaining definitions out of the way and explain exactly how these definitions are applied to taking your quest to free yourself from anxiety. It is my hope these explanations are able to shed a bit of light upon some of these concrete ideas on which this quest is based on.

Courage is Taking a Known Risk For a Known Reward

The theme of courage, much like in fictional stories of heroism, is a rather sizable aspect of your journey. Courage can be many things. Courage can be anything from telling someone how you truly feel about them, to finally going on a roller coaster you have been afraid to try out—in this case, courage is finally taking the steps long overdue to treat and permanently overcome your anxiety. On this quest, you will have to be prepared for the good, the bad, and everything in between. In fact, it is more likely you will be faced with a bit of a trial and error period, where you must try out a vast array of methods and techniques before being able to effectively determine what sticks best.

This means you will also have to take some unavoidable risks, which too, is a sign of courage. When put frankly, by pushing yourself to take risks and try new methods of treatment, which you know may not all be successful, you are exercising a marvelous feat of courage. This is predominantly because in deciding to take this kind of calculated risk, you are prioritizing the potential benefits that come from doing so over the consequences. In effect, this is a fundamentally positive approach to maintain while in your trial-and-error process, which is a fantastic way to stay motivated when the process gets a bit discouraging from time to time. In the context of this quest, one of the many ways your courage will shine through is by taking known risks for known rewards.

Sobriety

Many people, including yourself, are probably quite familiar with the word sobriety. Although sobriety is typically associated with abstinence from alcohol and other addictive substances, its meaning in the context of your quest is entirely different. Instead of working towards abstinence from alcohol and other addictive substances, the goal of your quest is to work your way towards sobriety from your anxiety.

When taking a step back to examine unmanaged anxiety on an abstract level, all it really is, is a nasty habit, or addiction, your brain has taken a firm hold of. As you have now learned from earlier chapters, experiencing feelings of anxiety only primes your brain to do it again more readily in the future. Eventually, your brain's anxious response becomes habitual, leaving you caught in a vicious cycle; much like having an addiction. Viewing your freedom from anxiety as sobriety is what makes the end goal of your quest both tangible and firm, and can definitely make accomplishing your goal feel much more rewarding.

Distinctions Between Anxiety and Fear

As part of the complicated nature governing human emotional responses, there can be a great deal of overlap between certain emotions—sometimes even to a point of one being misconstrued for another. This, at least in part, can be credited to the fact when we are experiencing one emotion, such as excitement, we are more likely to experience other emotions believed to be related to the initial emotion, such as happiness. This can be seen as both a good and a bad thing. Being able to experience more than one emotion simultaneously is a good thing because it speaks to how your development becomes far more complex with age, but at the same time, this convoluted mess of emotions can be very overwhelming at times and make it much more difficult to pick apart emotions behind an issue causing you distress. This is the very case when it comes to anxiety, as many people who are afflicted have a great deal of trouble picking apart their illness, largely due to the intricacy of what they feel when experiencing their symptoms. Because of this, it is important to your success that you learn how to identify the distinctions between anxiety and fear.

So what is the difference between these seemingly non-interchangeable terms? Well, in short, the largest difference between these two terms is the context in which they arise. While they without a doubt, do have overlap, the context of feeling anxious is usually in response to a threat anticipated, unanticipated, or not well defined. On the other hand, the context of feeling fearful is merely associated with a threat established and understood. What this means is, when you are experiencing an anxious response, even though the threat is not very well understood, your brain will nevertheless still try its absolute hardest to make sense of the situation.

However, because it is very difficult at the moment for your brain to produce an accurate assessment of the situation, the perceived threat can easily be exaggerated or excessive and elicit a fearful response. This resulting fearful response is usually extremely misguided, as people become convinced their loosely defined, disproportionate, irrational interpretation of a threat, is actually well understood and justified. Ultimately, the distinction is the real threat. When a gun is pointed at you, you are afraid a bullet will come out and harm you.

Anxiety is the same emotion, but there is no bullet, and being afraid is only in your head. Unfortunately, the difference is hard to determine at times, so during your first panic attack, you could end up going to the emergency room because it feels like you are having a heart attack. Having no other way of reassuring yourself what you feel is only in your head, not your chest.

The reason why fear and anxiety are often confused can primarily be attributed to the fact they both invoke similar stress responses. These stress responses are not necessarily a bad thing, however, as having the ability to activate a flight or fight response is important to your survival. Building off this, this means it is the event or situation that differentiates whether the stress response is triggered by fear or anxiety. Unlike fear, feelings of anxiety are accompanied by many more distressing symptoms. On top of this, anxiety can trigger your mind to run wild over the potential possibility of danger, rather than actual danger.

For example, an anxiety-based stress response would be feeling your palms start to sweat and your heart race before taking your turn to speak during a presentation. Even though the presentation poses no actual apparent threat, your body still produces a response more than likely to be confused with fear. From this, serious issues can arise because your stress responses can become increasingly more unreliable as your anxiety worsens to become chronicand or debilitating.

When looking at fear, by comparison, the stressors provoking true fear-based responses operate a bit differently. When it is fear, instead of anxiety, triggering the stress response, it is automatic and usually in response to a definite and dangerous threat, rather than a perceived one. In a situation where the threat is certain, stress-based responses are a proper reaction to being elicited by your body, to ensure your own survival. A fear-based stress response will always have a tangible stimulus triggering it—it is essentially your autonomic nervous system performing in situations where it is intended to. While it is true, a stress-based response, whether provoked by anxiety or fear, will result in physical symptoms automatically, it is only anxiety that brings about these symptoms as a result of a maladaptive assessment of danger in specific situations and circumstances.

LEFT OPEN FOR NOTES

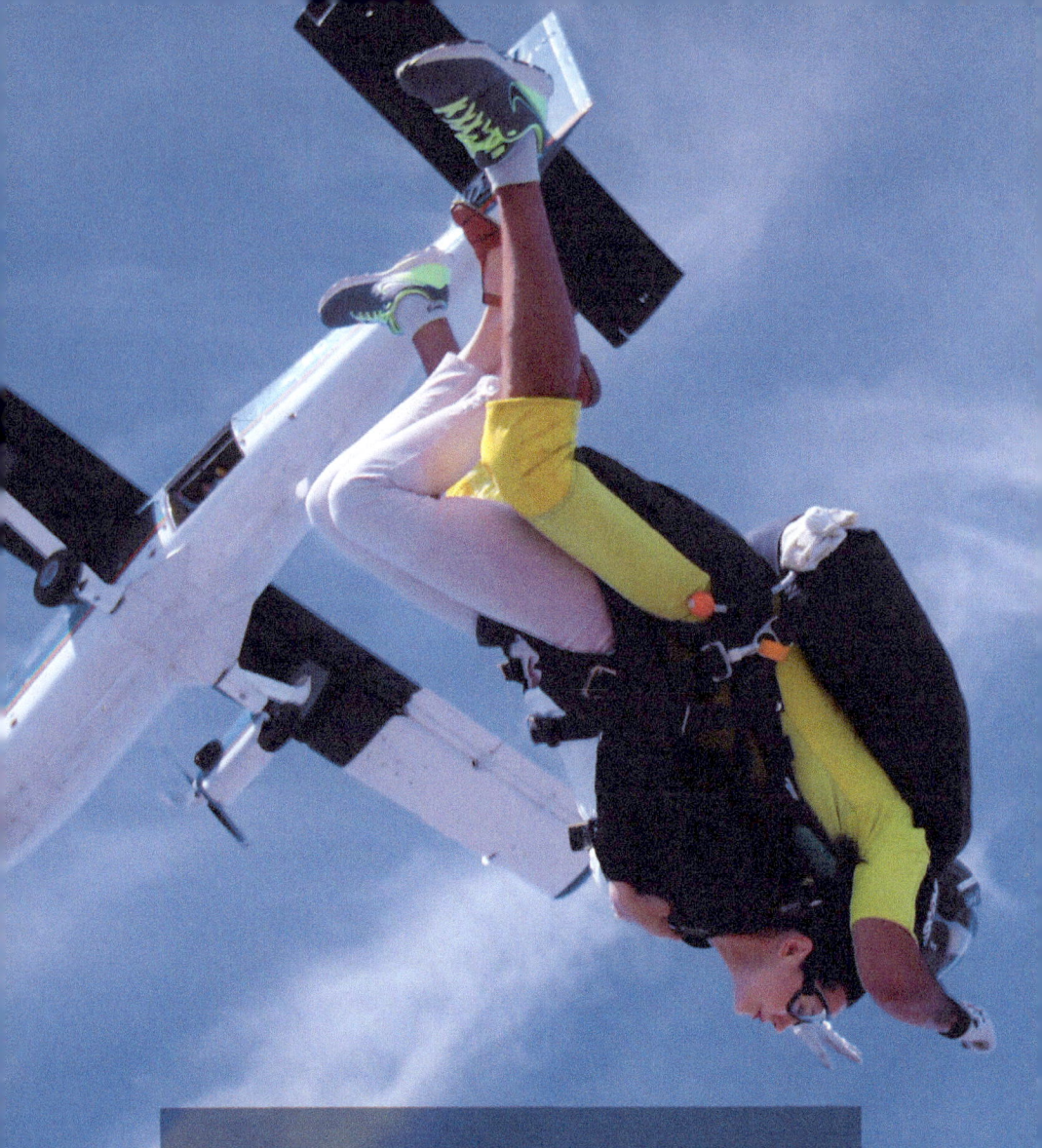

DEVELOPING COURAGE

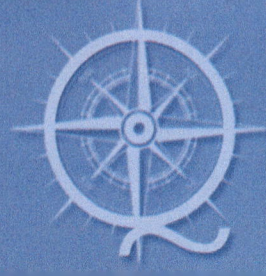

Chapter 3: Developing Courage

Courage, being the core of the drive needed to persevere no matter the circumstances, is a trait many people believe they lack. This is especially common with those of us who are afflicted with anxiety, who often feel as though we are powerless over our feelings and symptoms. In reality, this belief is far from the truth. Absolutely anyone, even those afflicted with anxiety, has the capacity to find and develop a sense of courage that guides them on their quest to anxiety sobriety. I can attest to this, through all of those whom I have helped over the years. In fact, one patient in particular, whom I worked with to build their courage, was a teacher whose performance anxiety was so severe it had prevented him from ever giving a speech during his entire life.

When I first met him, I had no doubt this patient loved his job as unconditionally as he loved his students. His biggest issue was, with the exception of speaking with children, he was completely and utterly petrified at the idea of speaking in front of any group. He even confessed he had managed to avoid any sort of situation throughout most if not all of his schooling, including grade school, college, and his masters. Any time a presentation or speech was assigned in the class he was in, he had always managed to renegotiate with his teachers and professors to let him do an alternative assignment not involving standing to present in front of his peers. This was unsurprising for me—public speaking is actually the number

"It's OKAY to be scared. Being scared means you're about to do something really, really brave." —Mandy Hale one fear reported on every anxiety survey conductedin America, so he was definitely in good company!

He was a smart man; he knew quite well how irrational it was to fear things like cancer, car accidents, and COVID, less than the simple act of speaking in front of his colleagues. Yet, he couldn't bring himself to overcome the potential, but unlikely negative reactions of his audience. His breakthrough, ironically, came from taking the opportunity to look at his performance anxiety from a different perspective. He understood his anxiety was rooted in his concern over how he would do and whether he would fall short of his audience's expectations, which he believed would result in disappointment, failure, and criticism. He got over this irrational concern, however, by realizing the people in which he was presenting in front of, were keen to hear what he had to say and had no intention of being critical or rejecting him.

So when he finally resolved to give a speech at the start of the following school year, he practiced fervently in front of his friends, knew the content he would be saying impeccably, and pictured his idealized end in mind, which was his co-workers, students, and peers gratuitously patting him on theback. To his excitement, his method worked! He had successfully and seamlessly delivered his speech and credited his success to his focus on his supportive audience and the important content they wereeager to hear. Because of his focus, he managed to avoid any feelings of nervousness or dry mouth,which were the usual symptoms plaguing him at even just the thought of speaking publicly. Through his concentrated efforts and willpower, he had successfully managed to build the courage he needed to complete his journey and overcome his anxiety to regain the self-confidence to keep him fearless, like in his childhood.

My patient's story is just one of the thousands of people who were able to find the courage toovercome their anxiety. With the right effort and resources, this can truly be possible for anyone to accomplish this feat; be willing to stay on the path of your quest no matter what is thrown your way. As explained in 2 Timothy 1:7, "For God has not given us a spirit of fear and timidity, but of power, love, and self-discipline."

To help you with this, the rest of this chapter is dedicated to teaching all the ways you can build your sense of courage to face your fears, feel your emotions, finish the impact of your past, forgive yourself and everyone involved, and finally accept where you have been, where you are, and where you want to be. Learning how to build the courage you need to address all of these things, will be of great asset to you in accomplishing the final goal of your quest—sobriety from your anxiety.

To Face Your Fears

There are several ways in which you can build the courage to face your fears. Learning how to face your fears is a very important tenet in overcoming anxiety, as much of the time people who are afflicted with anxiety must learn how to confront what stirs fear within them in order to determine the best method to treat it. I realize this is much easier said than done, so the purpose of this section is to give you a few examples to help you build the courage to face your fears.

The method my patient, the teacher, used is a perfect example of a very feasible method to help with building courage: imaging the alternative outcome of your anxiety-inducing situations.

For a moment, try to imagine the result of always letting your fear win, living a life ruled by fear and paralysis. Not only will the cost of letting your fear control you become much more of a reality to you, but it will also give you a bit of perspective when thinking next about what your life could be like if you didn't allow it to be ruled by fear. In doing so, you should be able to identify a stark difference between you controlling your fear versus your fear controlling you. In the case of the teacher, he utilized diligent practice and mindset, to imagine a situation where he had already successfully given his speech, which led to his success. Ultimately, every choice you make is yours, but fear does not improve without the motivation or willpower that works to overcome it.

One of the best ways to build the courage to overcome your fears is to rationalize them. When feeling fearful, logic is not usually something present, as it is only natural to act on instinct when faced with distressing circumstances. Similar to the previous method mentioned, the key part to all of this is putting things into perspective. Try thinking about a situation typically triggering you, but without pushing yourself too hard as to invoke an actual anxious response. Write a list of the worst things possible to realistically happen in this situation, should you have to actually ever endure it.

Doing this is a great way to help you look at a situation usually triggering you, at more of a face value, and help you think more rationally about whether your initial assessment of the posed threat was truly accurate. You can also use this method as a thought exercise to practice facing your fears until you feel as though you have built up the courage to do so for real.

Finally, learning to let go of things and circumstances you cannot control, is a very valuable trait to build upon and make facing your fears a much less painful process. Learning to let go is one of the hardest things to learn to do, to be able to grow as an individual and defeat personal challenges.

When you learn to let go, however, compartmentalizing your fears becomes a straightforward task.

There is no way you will ever be able to be completely in control of everything in your surrounding environment, but you will always be able to have full control over how you react to it. Learning to desensitize yourself to safe situations that produce a nonsensical fearful response, can really help with controlling your fears permanently.

There is no point in trying to plan for all the things that can possibly happen to you, as you go about your daily life, it is best to learn to go with the flow and take things as they come. You will likely find in doing so, a natural sense of courage will develop, as you become more confident in your ability to manage your reactions to situations on the fly.

To Feel Your Emotions

Managing emotions, when afflicted with anxiety, can feel much like a highly draining responsibility at times, which usually leads too many people merely choosing to bottle up their emotions instead of choosing to let them run their course. This is in no way healthy and is frankly just a recipe for disaster. Bottling up your emotions instead of learning how to navigate them, significantly increases the chance of having an emotional breakdown in the future. Building the courage to feel your emotion is something that takes time to do but is a lifelong skill that will help you with living a sustainable life, where you are in tune with how you truly always feel. There are a few ways you can learn to do this.

Learning to be confident in yourself while staying connected to others is how you can learn to make your decisions with more certainty and develop a better understanding of why and how some situations make you react more negatively than others. Understanding your emotions makes it far easier to allow yourself to feel them, which is why staying connected to others can really aid you with this endeavor. Relationships with others are how you can see and learn contextually about the emotions of others, which reflectively can help you in your analysis of your own. This also helps with building an intuitive sense, which too can be an arbitrating factor in emotional assessments.

Emotional intelligence is experiencing and expressing your feelings in healthy ways, then taking your response-ability to do something positive with your feelings. If you are anxious, notice it, use your ability to make a healthy response. Interpersonal emotional intelligence is similar to intrapsychic EI, becoming aware of what others are feeling, then responding appropriately to them.

In addition to this, keeping a big picture mentality and forcing yourself out of your comfort zone can build emotional resilience and help with putting your emotions into perspective, which can make big emotions seem much smaller and more manageable. Putting yourself into emotionally uncomfortable situations is sometimes what you need in order to mature your emotional intelligence. In doing so, it can help you realize just how much your anxious responses are an overreaction to the triggering situation and avoidance is not sustainable in the pursuit of looking to live life to the fullest. As stated before, learning to do this will take a great deal of patience and time but should be viewed as one of the many moving parts your success on this quest depends on.

To End the Impact of Your Past

Building the courage to end the impact of your past is a wildly important facet of your quest to sobriety from anxiety. By addressing the impact of your past, you are taking accountability and promoting mediation—both of which are essential to maintaining a realistic approach needed for your quest. There are many ways to learn to do this, but what works best for you is very dependent on your feelings towards your past, as some of us are more uncomfortable confronting past experiences we have pushed aside more than others. Either way, the two things I recommend to anyone who is faced with anxiety are learning to welcome failure and celebrating all courageous actions, no matter how big or small.

As an example, I'm so grateful you never heard me learning to speak English, Spanish, French, Vietnamese, Greek, or Hebrew because my many failures would have cost me some credibility in your mind. Maybe your failures were similar to my children's, like calling me "Dada" at first, which was music to my ears, not a catastrophic failure to use proper English. Anything worth doing, is worth doing poorly at first, even anxiety sobriety.

Confronting the past can be a very uncomfortable thing to have to do, mostly because for many it involves having to revisit failure. It has become much of an American cultural standard to fear failure—which has led to an over-anxious population as a result. By learning to accept failure, you are teaching yourself to adopt a more realistic perspective on your abilities and your limits. In addition, you will be able to recognize your growth from your failure, which would not otherwise be possible without reflecting back to see how far you have come. Can you remember your first attempt at skipping, hula hoop, riding a bike without training wheels, or even driving on the freeway? You have already accomplished overcoming many failures, all while learning to achieve success.

Building your courage is perfectly acceptable to do in increments; if anything, I would recommend it. This way, your progress is far more concentrated and paced, and is much more likely to be lastingand genuine. It is important to always celebrate the small accomplishments or benchmarks you reach when building confidence because this can serve as a motivator to continue working your way towards your goal, which is now closer than it was before. Praise your progress. Waiting for perfection will not work for you. Your courage in the future will always be worth more than your failure in the past. You are able to build the courage to end the impact of your past by celebrating your growth and keeping the mindset you will only move forward in the future.

To Forgive Yourself and Everyone Involved

Learning how to move on from feelings of resentment, to welcome feelings of forgiveness is vital to your ability to move on from your anxiety. The only way you will truly find fulfillment on this quest is by understanding not only is this a learning process for you, but it probably is for many of those around you as well. Learning to forgive others, especially in the case where you feel as though they wronged you, or were insensitive in some way to your struggles as a person afflicted with anxiety—will help you with becoming a more easy-going person, as well as help you accept situations at face value for what they are. After all, it is more than likely, much like yourself, these people had no tools or assets needed to help you mediate what you were going through and therefore were lost in regards to what actions to pursue to actually be helpful.

Everyone makes mistakes, and if you were to try and look at things from their perspective, you would probably see how much these individuals in your life actually care deeply about your personal wellbeing and want nothing but the best for you. In fact, conduct a survey with people who love you and ask them.

Circumstances and situations influence you and others more than you probably already believe. Humans are social creatures —much of the behavior we exhibit is modeled after other humans, who are just as likely to be confused by ambiguous or not well-defined circumstances as you are. The blame should not be shifted towards yourself or your peers, as in most cases of mental illness, it is unlikely most people involved had any sort of bad intentions with their interactions.

To practice forgiveness for yourself as well as others around you for the past you cannot change, I recommended you engage in the steps of accepting responsibility, accepting the remorse coming with stability, repairing the damage, and restoring the trust in yourself and your support system around you, and finally focus on renewal or moving forward onto bigger and better things.

Following these four steps can help you greatly with coming to terms with past experiences and memories where you must forgive yourself or others for their actions or lack of loving actions. Your journey to sobriety from anxiety is predicated somewhat on your ability to let go and forgive your past in order to experience the growth needed to complete the journey in full. Practice: look in the mirror and say, "I forgive you!"

To Finally Accept Where…

As has been reiterated many times throughout this book so far, all of the steps you have committed to taking in order to conquer your anxiety can very much be interpreted as a journey in which you are always looking to progress further on. The act of constantly moving forward is not usually something you can just "do" however. To execute this consistent progress successfully, you need to accept your past, your current circumstances, and finally have a clear set goal of where you want to be by the end of your quest. Taking the time to accept your past will help you with never being held back by your past regrets or guilty feelings. Acceptance doesn't mean you like the past and hope everyone has the same pain. To accept is to admit the truth, acknowledge reality, and acquire a life free of denial.

Establishing where you are currently on your journey helps you develop a realistic sense of what exactly progress has looked like so far, and determining where you want to be will help you with staying motivated as you move closer and closer to your goal of being anxiety-free.

The winter Olympics is happening as I write this. Do you accept every athlete has failed in the past? Do you admit they look anxious before their events? Do you acknowledge going fast on ice and snow in the past resulted in failures and pain? Do you believe if they can set and reach their goals, you can too, even if you have been anxious in the past? I do.

You've Been

Building the courage to come to terms with where you have been prior to starting, and in the earlier stages of this journey serves a few functions. First and foremost, doing this self-analysis of the exact areas you are looking to improve on during this quest can help significantly with mediating your past guilty feelings, or resentment over how you and others have handled certain situations in the past. In addition to this, you can more easily determine the baseline you started from, which is a great way to examine how you used to handle situations spiking your anxiety in the past, versus how you do so now in the present.

You Are

Building the courage needed to finally accept where you are on this quest can help you develop your sense of reality and what exactly you can accomplish when taking your journey day by day. You will probably surprise yourself and find you are actually far more capable than you previously believed, and have actually come very far from where you once were when you initially pursued this quest. You are a resilient, strong individual—and this is something I know I can say for sure, as everyone who is afflicted with anxiety is faced with the daily challenges of life to a much more severe degree than the average person. Your character sets you and others like you apart!

You Want to Be

Finally, you always want to be picturing the end of your journey finishing with great success. To do this, you must keep your goal in sight, make benchmarks at new milestones on this quest, and try to be cognizant, taking in as much as you can during each step along the way. Staying motivated is a key factor to constant progress, and once you have found the courage to finally accept where you have been in your past, where you are currently, and where you want to be in the future—you have created a highly personalized framework to follow in order to find your sobriety from anxiety forever.

LEFT OPEN FOR NOTES

FEELING CALM

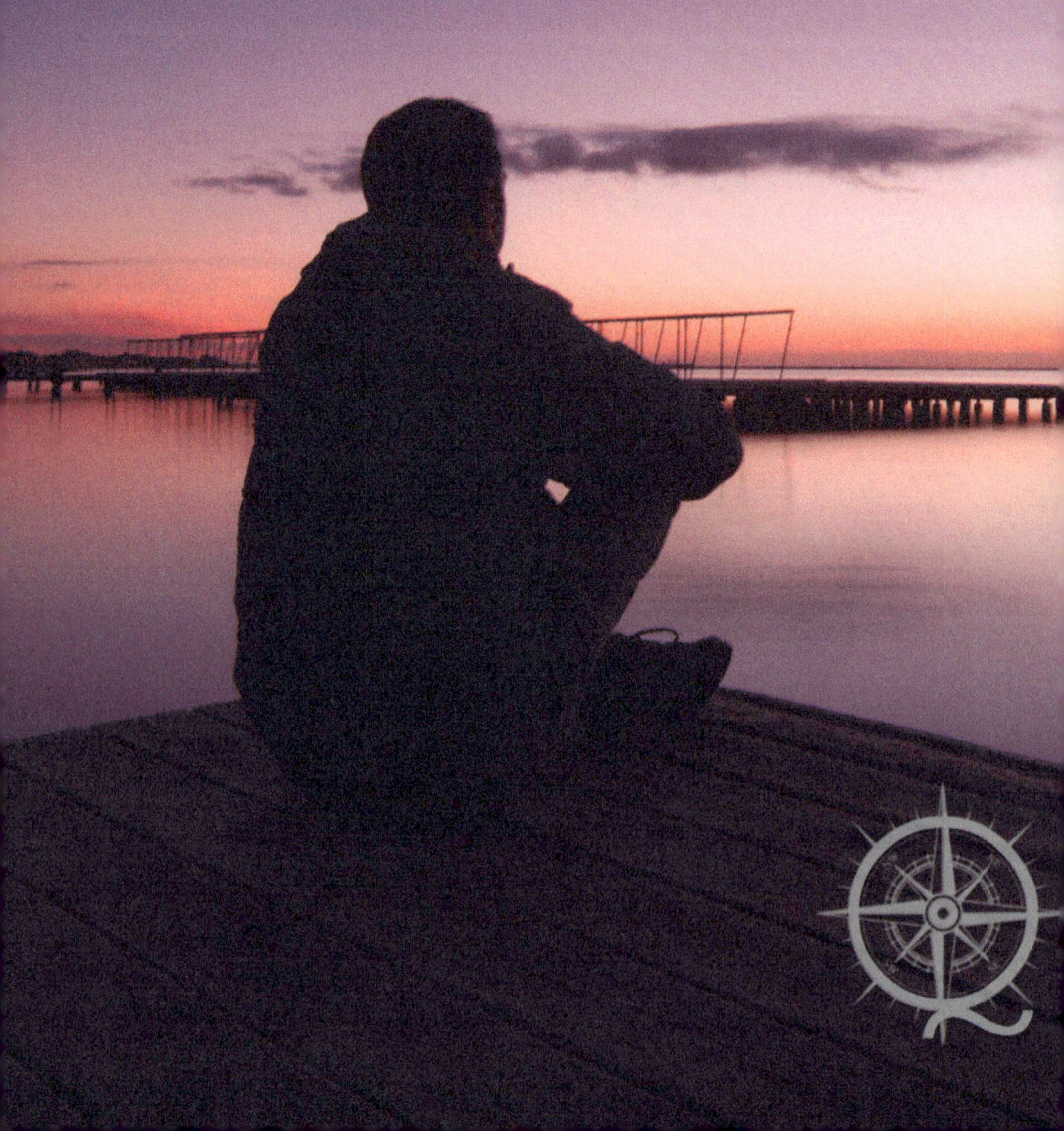

Chapter 4: Feeling Calm

Keeping an inner balance, otherwise known as maintaining your cool when a situation can spark anxious feelings, is a skill highly useful when learning how to control your symptoms and anxiety-based stress responses. There is simply no use in losing your cool—it will get you nowhere and do nothing but leave you feeling frustrated and out of control of your life. The good news is, this is definitely something you can learn to do, as even people who are not afflicted with anxiety can struggle from time to time with finding the calm feelings needed to rationally navigate a situation. To build upon this skill, however, you need to take the time to examine many different styles of coping mechanisms, and ways in which you can personally counteract symptoms of anxiety and panic where an anxious response is far from an appropriate reaction, given the situation or circumstance.

In addition to this, you can learn how you can identify your triggers, which is a task tricky to navigate, especially for those who have an anxiety disorder such as post-traumatic stress disorder, which can be debilitating when a flare-up of symptoms are experienced. However, simply knowing what your triggers are is a factor with a great deal of control over the intensity of your reaction and symptoms, so learning how to mediate, workaround or desensitize yourself to the triggers when you have identified them can work leaps and bounds in your favor. Also, it promotes constant progress, which is a fantastic motivator, as this quest to sobriety can be a long road to take, especially when you feel as though you still have a

"I promise you nothing is as chaotic as it seems. Nothing is worth diminishing your health. Nothing is worth poisoning yourself into stress, anxiety, and fear." – Steve Maraboli long way to go before you will be able to reach anxiety sobriety.

Problems With Panic

To feel calm when we are in a frightening situation is both difficult and enviable. We envy Batman, James Bond, and every character who gets out of a frightening time using the perfect gadget. We especially envy their ability to remain calm. However, in reality, the fight or flight chemicals wash over our frontal lobes where ordinarily we solve problems. Frightening situations produce more cortisol and less ability to use our tools effectively, meaning we sometimes lose our ability to rationally remain calm.

In 1978, I was ordained as the pastor of Grace Presbyterian Church in San Antonio. I was 26. The median age of the congregation was 76. The confidence needed to walk into the pulpit and preach to people the age of my grandparents was difficult and I was not feeling calm about it. However, before I preached my first sermon there, I used a tool in my faith: serve others and focus on them. The congregation had come to have a moment with God, not judge my performance.

Focusing on them, what God might say to them through me and my study of the Bible passage, helped me feel excited, not panic-stricken. Compassion for them, not my brain or its fight or flight chemicals, is what gave me the confidence to preach. Have you noticed when you are anxious you are focusing on yourself?

Feeling calm while preaching to people so old and wise, could have been terrible. The simple gadgetof unselfishly focusing on what I could give quieted any fright. One reason why public speaking is always reported as the number one anxiety in the US is it usually leads to you focusing on yourself instead of the listener. To feel calm by serving someone more anxious than you will help the speaker and listener.

Letting those intense feelings of panic take over in a time of crisis, instead of taking a step back to take a breath and look at the situation more realistically, is just one of the many problems with panic. Panic clouds your judgment, which is more than likely to result in a domino effect getting worse andworse the longer it goes without any sort of preventative intervention. Panic does nothing but makeeverything worse, so learning how you can personally counteract it when you feel the symptoms coming to head will help you in the long run.

The methods you will find to be the most useful in reducing panic and increasing calm, are ones you can use for the rest of your life. It is highly unlikely once you figure out what works for you, after reflecting on your anxiety and dissecting it enough you understand the roots and details of it, you will ever need to seriously alter these methods.

Allowing panic to exercise the degree of control it does, is to actively shoot yourself in the foot. I am sure you, as the person affected with anxiety, know just how much panicking can interrupt your daily life and prevent you from completing what you need to get done. This in effect also disrupts your potential for exponential development, leaving you stagnant as though you are fighting a battle that you will never be able to win.

No one deserves to feel helplessly vulnerable, but the only person who can really make a difference in minimizing or eradicating these feelings is you and the action you take. You will only be free fromyour problems of panic and therefore be able to accomplish your sobriety from anxiety once you have learned how to address your anxiety with potent methods and tips you have discovered through your own research, trial, and error.

Solutions to Panic Attacks

Maybe you are one of the people affected with anxiety and are subject to physical symptoms leading to panic attacks if the stimulus is severe enough. The best place to start is to identify your triggers and know what you can do to counteract panic attacks when a trigger is unavoidable or inevitable.

Before sharing the tips, methods, and techniques to help you in this endeavor, it is best to clarify two misconceptions about panic attacks. First, experiencing panic attacks as a response to a triggering stimulus does not make you an insane, absurd or lesser person by any means. Panic attacks and symptoms of anxiety are your body's method of release when under a great deal of stress, and are quite literally impossible to control without having the proper knowledge or skill set to do so.

Secondly, because panic attacks are a symptom of fierce, untreated anxiety, just knowing what your triggers are and how to calm yourself down during a panic attack is not enough to stop panic attacks from happening ever again. You must also learn how to break down your anxiety for what it is and be working towards addressing it, as you need to address the root cause to truly put it to an end. The last thing you want is for your anxiety to turn into an actual panic disorder, which is the next step anxiety progresses towards when it is not properly or fully treated.

Discovering your triggers and which methods work best for keeping you calm means you must be willing to put yourself in situations where you are exposed to your triggers, so it is important not to overexert yourself because this can disrupt your progress and push you beyond your limits, which can be a serious demotivator and throw you wildly off course.

Identifying Triggers

When breaking down how to find working solutions to minimize your panic attacks, a fundamental tenet of doing so involves identifying your triggers. Again, this is a key part of this process mostly because your triggers are the initial indicators of what causes you to feel the anxiety symptoms you do. A noteworthy way to do this is to take the time to write out how you feel in the moment while experiencing it. In addition, explore abstract situations you have concluded lead to you feeling anxious.

By keeping a journal of sorts, you are making the task of self-reflection much easier, which can make dissecting your anxiety to determine all of its pieces second nature. In a similar vein, by keeping a record of your symptoms as well as the times and settings in which you typically feel them, you can successfully isolate the stressors and triggers in your life that aggravate your anxiety and determine how you can take steps to improve both.

However, I recognize writing is not for everyone, as some people have trouble remembering or bringing themselves to transcribe how they feel in situations they find make them anxious. If you find you relate to this, I would recommend looking to a trusted person in your life whom you can talk to about these triggering situations and circumstances. This person can be absolutely anyone including a religious leader, a licensed clinician, a friend, a loved one, or even a community leader. What is of the highest importance in choosing to do this is you have full trust in the person you have chosen to speak with and are willing to share everything you need to about your struggles with anxiety. On top of this, by choosing to talk to a person, you can also provide yourself the opportunity, if you are comfortable enough, to address potential previous trauma you believe could contribute to your triggers or act as a trigger itself.

Lastly, make a point of trying to listen to your body. The amazing thing about the human body is it will actually inform you of whether it approves of what you are doing or not, in one way or another.

Since sugar is a very big player in the game of making the most of your brainpower, staying mindful of your diet, especially when ingesting food and drinks known to not be great for your health, is one of the easiest ways you can ensure the anxious symptoms you feel are not being exacerbated by other controllable factors. You may even find certain food or drinks are a trigger for you, which is ideal not only because it kills two birds with one stone, but also because a trigger of this type is one of the easiest to control and work around. Identifying a trigger of this sort can also act as a motivator to continue working to determine what the rest of your triggers are because you will realize figuring out one trigger makes you closer to putting an end to your panic attacks than you were previously.

Preventing Panic Attacks

It may feel impossible to you at this point, but there are many ways your anxiety can work towards preventing panic attacks even in the most triggering of situations. It is important to not underestimate just how effective having a proper skill set to do this can be. Knowing how to do this will always be an asset in a time of crisis. This being said, you must also take care of yourself in a general sense in order to make the most out of counteractive techniques and methods.

Maintaining your physical and mental health outside of your anxiety actually has a bigger effect than you realize, and can act as a silent culprit preventing you from continuous progress. As you read through these suggested tips and methods, consider how well you take care of yourself by eating healthily, getting enough sleep and exercise, reducing your caffeine intake, and engaging in relaxation techniques.

Aside from the physical maintenance, you should be keeping up with, putting work into having a good mindset is also an important thing that makes a big difference in eliminating panic attacks. The use of various kinds of relaxation techniques, such as meditation, yoga, deep breathing, and massage, are all quite straightforward yet highly effective in cultivating a good mindset. Sometimes, learning to accept you will not be able to control everything you come across, while difficult, can be rewarding when accomplished. This is because doing so once again reinforces that letting go is one of the most effective ways to stay grounded and you will only ever be able to be in full control of how you react to situations.

Maintaining this kind of mindset teaches you there is nothing to lose, as you are only a person who can do so much. As a result, this kind of mindset marvelously complements the act of challenging any intrusive thoughts you may have as triggers for your anxiety. If you never learn to challenge these intrusive and triggering thoughts, letting go becomes a far more arduous task than it needs to be.

Using breathing is one of the chosen relaxation techniques that can make a big difference when trying to calm down. A technique widely recommended and used is called the 4-7-8 breathing technique. To properly execute this technique, you take a deep breath, inhale for four seconds, hold your breath for seven seconds, and exhale slowly for eight seconds. The use of this technique can behighly effective when looking to prevent hyperventilation during the onset of symptoms. By timing your breathing, you are able to distract your mind from the triggering stimulus onto something else that is simple to keep up with, but also effective enough to keep your mind away from an anxious response. However, if you find deep breathing techniques, such as this one, only make your symptoms worse as you begin to feel your anxious response kick in, it is recommended you consider alternative methods of panic attack prevention.

Another great technique to help with refocusing yourself to become grounded is called the 5-4-3-2-1 method. This kind of technique is based on mindfulness, which is a very salient concept in the event of needing to calm down from a climbing panic attack. This method consists of five steps. Remember it is important to not rush when applying this method as its effectiveness depends on you taking your time to ensure you are making the most of each step, which in turn will reap the greatest reward by the end.

First, look around in your environment and choose five different objects, taking the opportunity to think about what each object is or what purpose they serve. Next, try listening closely to your surrounding environment and see if you can pick out four distinct sounds. Once you have chosen your sounds, try thinking about what makes each sound different so you can pick it apart from others. You can even rate the sounds by how much you like or dislike them—the idea behind this exercise is there is ample flexibility in what you choose to focus on, so it can be adapted to what you are capable of doing at any moment in time.

Once you have identified and thought about sounds, try and find three individual objects you can touch. These can be the exact same objects you identified during the first step of this technique if you happen to be somewhat limited by your environment, or they can also be entirely new objects. While you are taking the time to touch the objects you found, think about some of the properties of the objects such as how they feel in your hands as you hold them.

Next, take a whiff of the air around you and try to identify two separate smells. These smells can be anything, such as the smell of gasoline from the cars on the street, or the scent of the perfume you sprayed on yourself before leaving the house. Finally, if you are in an environment where it is possible, see if you can find a food item or drink you can ingest so you can engage the last of your senses, taste. This can be any food or drink, but it is recommended you choose something interesting, not inoffensive in flavor or texture.

This technique has grown wildly in popularity due to its magnitude of effectiveness in grounding uswhen we feel panic symptoms. The reason behind its effectiveness is when executed correctly, it requires us to completely disrupt the mindset allowing for the symptoms of a panic attack to develop. By engaging all five senses, we are allowing ourselves to find balance through the use of our surrounding environment and realistically ground ourselves.

If you know for certain breathing techniques do not worsen your symptoms, the use of the 4-7-8 breathing technique can also be used in this technique and combined with the step where you must identify smells. Not only will you be breathing deeply, which promotes calming down, but doing so can potentially make this technique even more effective for you and get you closer to the baseline you are trying to reach much faster.

Daily routines are also super useful for those who experience panic attacks as a result of their anxiety. A routine minimizes the chance of an unanticipated situation, which is usually the cause of mostphysical symptoms from anxious responses. A routine will make you comfortable, and create a setting where you feel as though you have the headspace to engage in some deep reflection about your anxiety and why it has the capacity to elicit such a vicious stress response. Routines will make successfully getting through the daily challenges you usually face a regular habit and give you a bit more control over your circumstances. If you feel as though it would help you, this daily routine can even include making a schedule to plan your day so you can avoid feeling unnecessarily anxious at any point in your day.

However, if you feel as though busying yourself to prevent ruminating on your anxiety will make things worse, choosing points in your day to allow yourself to feel your anxious feelings for a set period of time may be the dose of catharsis you really need to keep moving forward. If you are not too keen on following routines, another great technique is to actively put yourself in situations or circumstances in which you are positive you enjoy, such as engaging in hobbies, hanging out with close friends, or volunteering. Doing activities and putting yourself in situations sparking your happiness is very important as well for finding the balance you need.

Should you feel as though a panic attack may be imminent no matter what method you try, there are steps you can take to minimize the emotional outburst. As you feel the climb building, see if you are able to isolate the primary thought racing through your mind when you typically experience a panic attack. Being able to successfully isolate thoughts fueling the vicious feedback loop, can help with alleviating common panic symptoms of helplessness or suffocation. Finding the focus to do this can be profoundly difficult, especially when a panic attack is near its summit, but this task can be significantly expedited by bringing your attention to a singular, unchanging attribute of the situation or circumstance.

An example of this would be staring at a stationary object or person, in close enough vicinity, so your focus allows you to tune out all of the other stimuli around you, and tune into your internal thoughts and feelings. In addition to this, if you believe it could be helpful in triggering situations, having someone whom you can go to, or can accompany you, in high-risk situations is a fantastic addition to the method. Having a buddy, or identified safe person, is a very fast and effective way to help distract you when you feel panic symptoms or need to leave a triggering situation without causing a scene.

In the same realm as using distractions to trick your brain, using a more difficult task such as counting backward from the highest number you can think of, with your eyes closed, is also a rapid way to counteract an oncoming panic attack. Engaging in a difficult task during the onset of your symptoms, like counting backward, can produce wildly successful results due to the fact the area of the brain propagating complex executive logic-based tasks has the capacity to override protractive emotional processes. This means with the right stimulus, at the right time, you can use a logical process to neutralize an emotional one and bring yourself back to the baseline you need to be at to make the right decisions and act accordingly, whether it be changing some triggering aspect of the situation or removing yourself from the situation entirely.

Finally, a quick useful tip you can take under consideration that helps with preventing a panic attack when you find yourself in a perceived threatening situation, is to look around your environment and see if you can identify all of the potential triggers in the setting, and how you can work around them. This way, you are putting a conscious effort into minimizing the chance of surprise encounters with potential triggers and therefore lowering your chances of actually having a disproportionate emotional response. Identifying your triggers can also help you realize nothing about the situation or circumstances you find yourself in is permanent, and this situation will without a doubt come to pass.

Tips for Coping

When looking for regular coping mechanisms to alleviate some of your anxiety, the great news is there are many, many different kinds of coping mechanisms—far too many to cover in just this section alone. Coping mechanisms are also extremely personal and in essence, can really be anything as long as it is not harmful to anyone around you or self-destructive to your wellbeing. For the sake of time, only a handful of the multitude of coping mechanisms will be shared in this section. The point of this is to help you generate some ideas of ways that help you cope, in addition to the coping mechanisms that are already widely used by many. You can cope with your anxiety by:

- Repeating self-affirming mantras

- Creating a routine you know stimulates you and calms you down
- Engaging in meditative practices such as mindful exercises, deep breathing, and yoga
- Determining a scent, sight, sound, taste, or touch you find is good at relaxing you when you feel anxious
- Finding a hobby to make you happy and takes your mind off things
- Speaking to someone whom you trust about what you are going through
- Practicing self-love and reflecting on all you have accomplished
- Creating an action plan of steps you know can bring you back to your baseline
- Spending time in nature
- Making time to spend quality time with loved ones and friends
- Learning to find the silver lining in negative situations where it feels as though everything is going wrong.

LEFT OPEN FOR NOTES

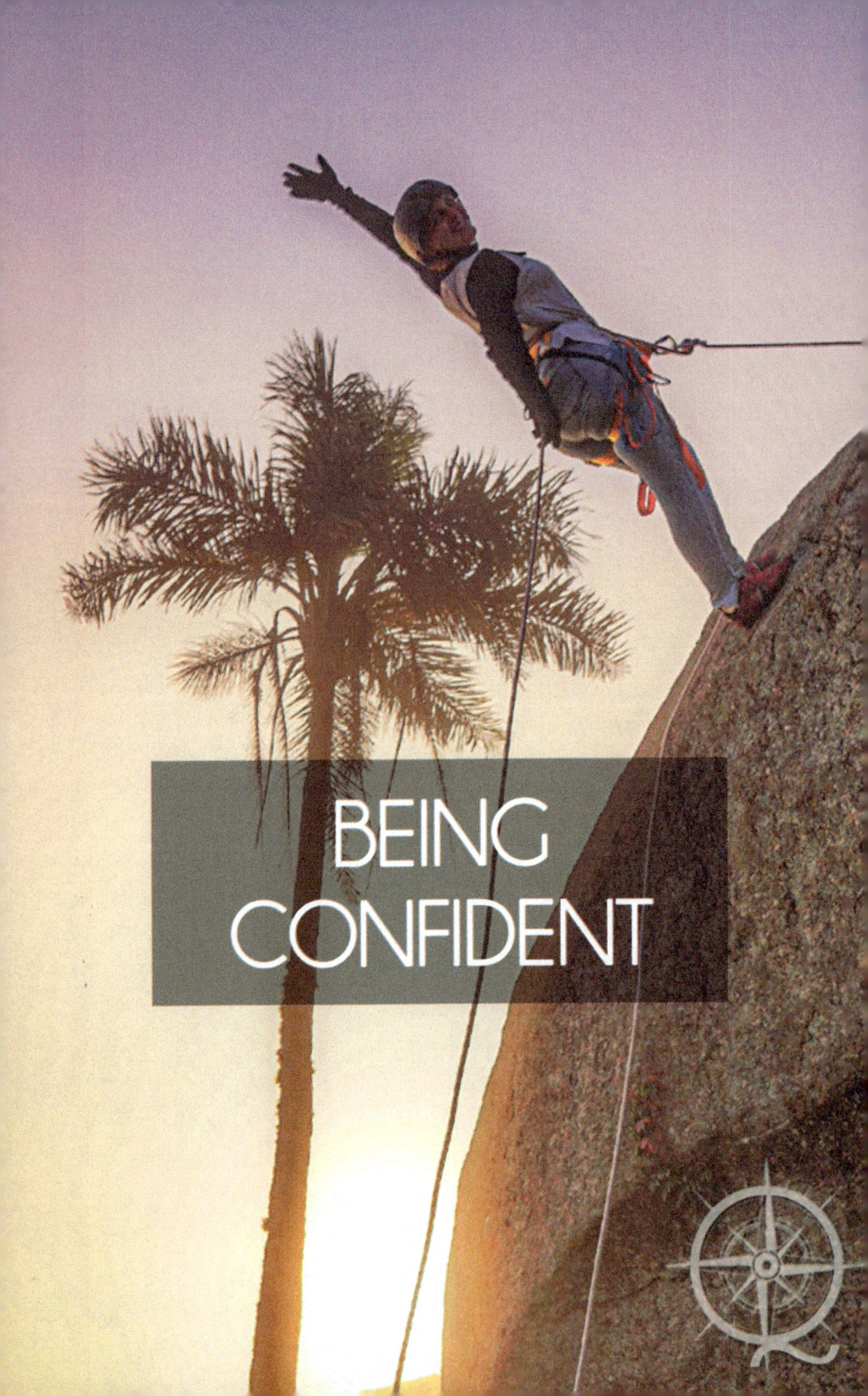

BEING CONFIDENT

Chapter 5: Being Confident

Among many of the things you need to be developed on this quest, confidence is one of the most broadly applied skills you will use. You probably grew up hearing phrases such as "confidence is key", which are often said to reassure those who are experiencing anxiety or a lack of self-assurance in something they are looking to accomplish. But saying you should be confident is far different from actually being a confident person. Confident individuals do not need to advertise the fact they are confident—they display they are through their actions and judgment, especially when they need to rely upon it the most. Similar to courage, confidence is a quality pretty much all heroes in fictional stories possess, especially in the stories of King Arthur and the Jedi. But once again, having this trait does not need to be limited just to fictional characters, it is attainable for anyone who puts their mind and best efforts towards it.

Usually, maybe you believe having anxiety is not conducive to building confidence, let alone being a confident person. This assumption is very incorrect, as even those with anxiety can achieve this feat and if anything, it is entirely necessary to do so in order to find your freedom from anxiety. The approach you take, however, is quite a bit different than the average person, as they must first build the courage needed to overcome their anxiety before even beginning to work on their confidence to continue and move forward. You are in no way tied to your insecurity for longer than you let yourself be, but for the patience required to pull yourself up and out of the

"You may not control all the events that happen to you, but you can decide not to be reduced by them."

– Maya Angelou

hole of insecurity, you become willing to fight against any feelings causing you to doubt yourself or the decisions you are making.

Problems With Nervousness

Nervousness, along with all the other physical symptoms of anxiety, can be a pesky aspect of physical anxiety that is hard to shake. Nervousness can cause you to trip up on your words, forget what you aresaying, make your legs shake, and your palms sweat, which can create a negative feedback loop where the more cognizant you become of your physical symptoms, the more nervous you feel. Sometimes, nervousness can outright prevent you from accomplishing something you have sought to do. But nervousness does not need to be the big, scary monster it is commonly made out to be. It is totally normal to feel nervous from time to time, but when it debilitates you, it is an increasing point of concern to really be addressed.

When you are nervous, you are much less likely to be thinking rationally about the situation or accurately assessing the perceived risks you believe are grounds to be feeling the way you do. The goal should always be to try and approach every situation with a calm mindset, as there is far more to gain from believing everything will go your way rather than falling to pieces. Nervousness is highly associated with specific kinds of anxiety such as performance anxiety, which has become all too common in our society today. By solving your problems with nervousness through isolating situations and circumstances making you anxious, you will be able to approach nerve-wracking situations with minimal symptoms, a clear head, and an open mind.

Performance Anxiety

At this point in the chapter, I feel as though it would be best to share an anecdote of another one of my patients who struggled deeply with performance anxiety. Years ago, this patient was an engineering student who decided to seek intervention for his performance anxiety during his junior year of college. He was a fantastic student, very intelligent, and was looking to land an internship as a part of his degree. He was a perfect student aside from his grades on presentations, where he would become so nervous he would be unable to perform to the best of his ability, despite knowing the content of his presentation and having prepared a great deal. Otherwise, he could remember anything he was taught in class or read in his textbook, so his inability to present often left him feeling frustrated and increasingly demotivated.

Together, we worked over time to alleviate his anxiety around presenting at school, and he eventually built the confidence necessary to overcome his uneasiness. He went his own way after this and I believed I had heard the last of him until he reached out again during his senior year to have some assistance in preparing for the important interview to determine whether he got the internship he had sought out. The stakes for this were much higher than presenting for school because he hoped he could be hired on for employment by the end of the internship. Once again, together we reframed his perspective on the interview from how badly he could blow it, to seeing himself answer the prayers of the company, their HR department, and the people interviewing him who would eventually become his coworkers. In the end, he managed to do an outstanding job during the interview and landed the internship. Hardly any of my patients call to check in once their treatment is complete, but he made a point of doing so, and we celebrated his joy and new mojo.

Solutions to Nervousness and Phobias

In order to get past all of your nervousness, it is important to learn about the different solutions that can greatly mediate the intensity of your symptoms or even ease them entirely. Similar to your anxiety, it is not the circumstances or situations making you nervous—you are a complex person with needs, hopes, wants, and dreams, but sometimes struggle with the self-confidence needed in order to get you there. However, as you have learned so far from this chapter, building the confidence needed to find solutions to your anxiety, nervousness, and phobias, is totally and completely possible with the right knowledge, effort, and dedication to your end goal. Two great methods to consider when thinking of solutions to curb your nervousness are using mindfulness and bodyfulness techniques, both of which will be explained further.

Mindfulness

You may or may not be familiar with the concept of mindfulness, but many people struggle to understand what it truly means to be mindful or how they can properly use mindfulness.

Mindfulness is the act of living in the present, existing as you are, and taking in everything around you. The purpose of mindfulness is to center you and bring you far back down to your baseline so you feel readjusted but also more connected to your internal processes and your external environment. Mindful- ness can also look like very many things: it can be anything from taking a few moments to yourself with your eyes closed to doing a yoga class in the morning when you wake up. Mindfulness, however, takes practice as it is free from judgment and you must have a clear mind while doing mindful exercises in order to make the most out of it. But if you are committed and happen to find a mindful exercise you enjoy, your motivation alone will develop your ability to do the technique very effectively in little to no time!

Bodyfulness

Bodyfulness, which is a proponent of mindful practice, is a group of techniques to make you more physically cognizant of how your body feels in a moment. Practicing bodyfulness can be even moreeffective than mindfulness, largely because a lot of the symptoms you face when triggered are physical in nature, rather than just psychological. Sometimes, when experiencing a physically anxious response, it can be easy to try and engage your body rather than your mind, and can also yield better results. Some recommended bodyfulness based exercises and techniques are pelvic floor, breathing 4by 4, and fingertip massage to yawn.

Pelvic Floor

This exercise is a very easy one to complete and only requires you to be able to stand in one spot. First, you must place one hand over your chest and the other over your stomach, right below your rib cage. Follow this step by taking a deep breath to a count of three, and then exhaling to a count of four. When you inhale, you are relaxing your pelvic floor, which then goes back to its resting statewhen you exhale. Do this exercise many times over, and slowly you will find yourself beginning to physically relax as you engage and disengage your pelvic floor. This exercise produces the best results when practiced daily for a few minutes at a time.

Breathing 4 by 4

Breathing 4 by 4, otherwise known as box breathing, is an easy breathing technique to apply at any moment while feeling unease symptoms. Box breathing should be done while sitting down, with your back supported and your eyes closed. First, you inhale through your nose while counting to four slowly, feeling the air enter your lungs. Next, hold your breath, without overexerting yourself, for a count of four seconds. Finally, exhale for four seconds and hold for another four seconds. This exercise should be repeated several times over several minutes in order to have the greatest effect.

Fingertip Massage to Yawn

Finally, try the fingertip massage to yawn, which is based slightly on acupuncture. You begin this exercise by massaging your fingertip on the side of your fingernail. By gently rubbing this pressure point, you can relieve a great deal of physical tension. Finish this exercise by stretching your arms up to induce a yawn, imagining the tension leaving from the tips of your fingers, to fully get rid of the tension you just pushed out of your system via your pressure point. This can be done on each fingernail until you feel you have released enough tension to bring you back to your baseline.

LEFT OPEN FOR NOTES

ACCEPTING FAILURE

Chapter 6:
Accepting the Consequences of Failure

Learning to accept the consequences of failure is a point reiterated throughout this book. Your past will always be a part of who you are, since it has shaped you to become the person you are today. So learning to accept your past, both the good and the bad, is important in the process of eradicating anxiety. For some people, a big source of anxiety comes from past negative experiences where you feel as though you could have acted differently or a negative situation caused issues you blame completely on you. While it may actually be the case you are valid in believing you could have handled a situation differently, there is no use in dwelling on it as nothing can be done to change the past. All you can do is forgive yourself and move forward.

Moving forward from this sometimes means having to accept the consequences of your previous actions, including past failures. This can also mean having to take accountability for things you have avoided addressing because doing so would result in putting you in an uncomfortable position—but this needs to happen while on your quest because you will never be able to accept how far you have come otherwise. You are able to fail and still accomplish fantastic things if you set your mind to it. When facing the consequences of your failure, try to remember your past transgressions do not mean they will be replicated in the future nor do they define your character.

"Do not let your difficulties fill you with anxiety; after all, it is only in the darkest nights that starsshine more brightly." – Ali Ibn Abi Talib

Freedom from anxiety is about accepting the circumstances and facing the music, even when it becomes a bit too much to bear.

Growth From Failure

On this journey, you will see by the end how much you have grown from your failures. Most people will fail many times over before finding success, and there is nothing wrong with failing. You should never fear failure, however; it is a vital aspect of your quest that helps you redirect when you have discovered a method you are trying is not working as well as you had believed it would. "Therefore do not fear them. For there is nothing covered that will not be revealed, and hidden that will not be known." - Matthew 10:26. What matters more than your failures, is your growth and how you apply growth to improve things for yourself.

Accepting your past is to accept the consequences of your previous failures, but also to recognize the benchmarks of your improvement over time. Your quest will build resilience and perspective within you; two qualities necessary when seeking to understand your growth from failure in the context of your journey to your sobriety from anxiety. This can even be applied if you are unsuccessful the first time around in your quest, which is entirely possible. You should not see this as a bad thing, however, now you know what does not work for you when attempting to treat your anxiety and there is no shame in starting again. You will never be alone in what you face, and your growth will always matter more than who you are or what you have done in the past when your doubt was out of control.

Alternative Forms of Treatment

When looking beyond coping mechanisms and all the various methods and techniques shared in this book, there are other forms of treatment and intervention you can utilize to help with alleviating your symptoms of uncertainty. Incorporating these forms of treatment is completely optional on this quest, but it is important to know about your alternative options should you find the resources you have selected for yourself are not doing enough to help you or are not quite the right fit for what you are looking to achieve. The two most common forms of alternative treatment not involving talk therapy or coping mechanisms are medication and the use of hotlines, helplines, and websites. Both of these alternatives can be highly effective, but there are pros and cons to both.

Medication

Medication, behind talk therapy and coping mechanisms, is a very common form of treatment usually incorporated when treating anxiety. The important caveat to consider with medication is it will not cure you. Medication for anxiety is only for treating your symptoms and is something you will likely have to keep up with daily. Medication must be used alongside other resources if you have the intention of curing yourself of your anxiety. Also, medication for anxiety is highly controlled as some kinds of medication are addictive.

This means in order to obtain a prescription for anxiety medication, you will get formally diagnosed with an anxiety disorder through a psychiatrist, which may or may not be too difficult of a process for you. Medication can have side effects potentially even worse than your anxiety when it goes on unmedicated, but a risk you might take when considering any form of medication for any ailment. When you find the correct medication and the correct dosage, medication can make a world of difference in treating suffering. Some commonly prescribed medications for anxiety include:

- Prozac
- Klonopin
- Zoloft
- Valium
- Xanax
- Librium
- Ativan

Hotlines, Helplines, and Online Resources

Choosing to use resources like hotlines, helplines, and online websites as a means of treating your anxiety is one of the most easily accessible ways to seek treatment. Fast and easy, you can talk to someone who is qualified to help you or find the information you are looking for in mere minutes.

The caveat of using these resources is it is a lot less personalized, so you may not be able to find the help you really need; the treatment makes a difference in how you handle your troubles.

If you are more just looking for general, unpersonalized but fast advice, there are many resources to choose from including:

- Psychguides.com
- National Suicide Prevention Lifeline: 1-800-273-8255
- Mentalhelp.net
- National Alliance on Mental Illness Helpline: 1-800-950-6264
- Teen line: 1-310-855-4673 or 1-800-852-8336

LEFT OPEN FOR NOTES

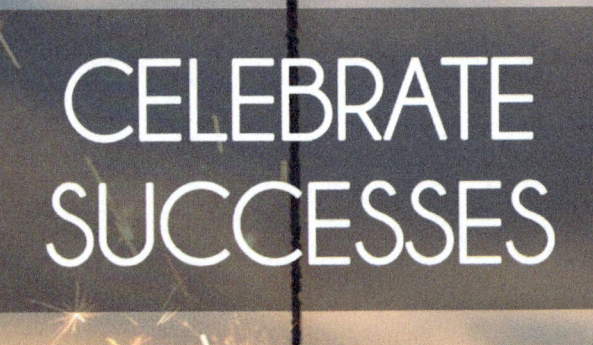

CELEBRATE SUCCESSES

Chapter 7:
Celebrating Your Successes

Once you have reached a certain point in your quest and you start to see clear progress from where you once began, it is important to celebrate. Celebrating your successes allows you the recognition you have both earned and deserve for all the hard work and effort in which you have put in toget you where you are. Think of the grand celebration ceremonies seen in movies such as Star Wars; brimming with happiness and recognition, the heroes of the journey receive the warranted praise they have eagerly awaited. While the celebrations you choose to partake in for your own successes need not be nearly as grand, you should nevertheless always acknowledge your progress in some shape or form.

Celebrating progress will keep you motivated to continue on to the end of your quest. Celebrating builds your confidence and courage. The journey you committed to taking is not easy by any means, no matter who tells you otherwise. Anxiety is a tough beast to fight off but with your dedication to psychoeducation, trial, and error, as well as an open mind, you have definitely put up a worthwhile fight thus far. Even in the case of experiencing a setback, it is important to stay mindful of the positives and what you have accomplished as opposed to what you have failed to accomplish. Your success is always worth celebrating because it is not only something you successfully did as the driving force, but it also puts into perspective all you are capable of doing when you set your

"All life is an experiment. The more experiments you make the better."
– Ralph Waldo Emerson

mind to it. By this point, sobriety from your anxiety feels as though it is just within arm's reach.

Recognizing What You Have Achieved

To recognize what you have achieved, take a step back and mentally review all of your past experiences and troubles you have faced on your journey. It is best to examine both your successes and your failures because it will then be more apparent to you how you used the assets you developed on this quest to work your way out of obstacles. In addition to this, you will get a strong sense of your ability to problem solve and remain strong through adverse times.

You deserve to treat yourself with love and respect, even if you have not completely gotten rid of your anxiety symptoms. The only person in this race is you, and the ribbon waiting for you at the end of the finish line will only be freshly broken when you cross it. You have come so far from who you once were when you let your anxiety take control of your life, and this should be readily apparent to you in your daily life and interactions with your external environment. The sky is your limit, but you have never actually stopped working your way up; so celebrate!

Complimenting Yourself

As a part of celebrating your successes, complimenting yourself is one of the easiest ways to celebrate. You deserve recognition for your hard work, as this is a very personal journey. Sometimes it is best for you to be the one giving the compliments to yourself. You are the one who is the most closely in tune with what you have accomplished. You are the only one who truly knows how hard you worked and how many sacrifices you made to get where you are today, therefore you are the only one who can give out compliments accurately reflective of your success. This form of self-love builds courage and confidence, which will always come to your aid while on this quest. After all, a great principle to always keep in mind is, "An anxious heart weighs a man down, but a kind word cheers him up." - Proverbs 12:25.

Famous People Who Have Overcome Anxiety

Anxiety may seem like a mental illness not really affecting prominent individuals within our society, but this could not be farther from the truth. Anxiety does not discriminate, there are several famous people and celebrities who have been afflicted and have had to learn to overcome their anxiety. Just like you, these celebrities worked hard to overcome distressing symptoms in certain situations and circumstances they had no control over. Some of these celebrities who have successfully taken their journey to earn sobriety from their anxiety include:

- TV host, Stephen Colbert

- Singer, Lady Gaga
- Reality TV star, Kim Kardashian
- Actress, Emma Stone
- Singer, Zayn Malik
- Former tennis player and current golfer, Mardy Fish
- And many more!

LEFT OPEN FOR NOTES

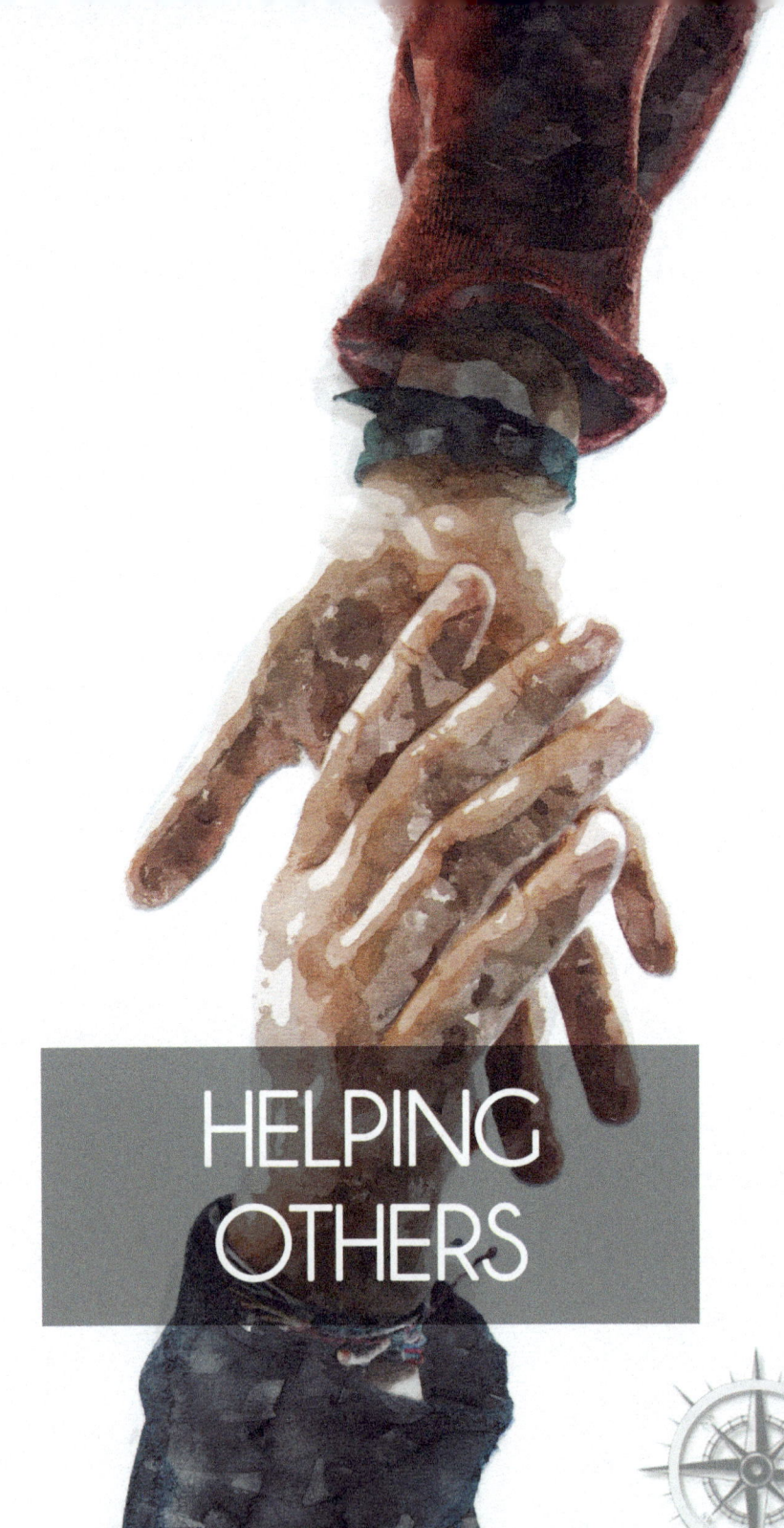

HELPING OTHERS

Conclusion: Helping Others with Anxiety

By the end of this long, intensive journey, you will likely be a brand new person. Now self-assured, confident, and courageous, you are ready to take on the world for what it is with an open mind and a relaxed demeanor. At this point, why not congratulate yourself for all you have done since you began this quest. Through all the ups and downs, you remained focused with your goal in sight, driving you to eventually reach the end. You took the time to educate yourself, take risks, develop your skillset, and find what treatment works best for you, which ultimately has led you to the success you have accomplished today.

You now have a very developed understanding of how unsustainable living a life riddled with anxiety actually was and managed to improve your circumstances for the better, all through sheer willpower. So now, it is time to move on with your life and spread your knowledge to help those who were once as anxious as you were; "Give to the one who asks you, and do not turn away from the one who wants to borrow from you."- Matthew 5:42. Just by lending an ear or spreading the information on the steps you took, you are making a marked difference in helping others with their anxiety.

Using your sobriety as an example can show others afflicted with anxiety they can do something to change how they are

"If you can't fly then run; if you can't run then walk; if you can't walk then crawl, but whatever you do you have to keep moving forward."
– Martin Luther King Jr.

feeling and if they work hard enough, they may be able to reach sobriety from their anxiety as well. You too can now attest to the fact managing your anxiety is to understand it, and you now have all of the skill set necessary to help others accomplish this as well. So now, the choice is yours—you realized through reading this book the right time to start working toward eliminating anxiety is now, and now it is your duty to instruct others on how to do the same in their quest.

Epilogue

Having now finished this book, it is time to address the So What and the What Now questions for readers like you. If you do have questions, you are probably thinking right now, "The book was helpful, but now I need Dr. Ray to help me with …":

- Coaching programs to build on my strengths
- High impact programs to learn more skills and tools
- Counseling to overcome mental health disorders
- Intensives in Spokane to make a lot of progress in a short time
- Intensives in your own town bringing in Dr. Ray to have help close by you

Any of these concerns you may find yourself having after having read this book, I am more than happy to lend a hand. Together, we can work to strengthen your mental fortitude and learn how to live your life to the fullest, where you control your mental illness rather than letting it control you!

LEFT OPEN FOR NOTES

EXTRA EQUIPMENT

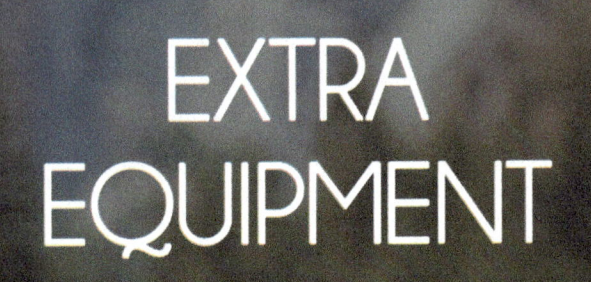

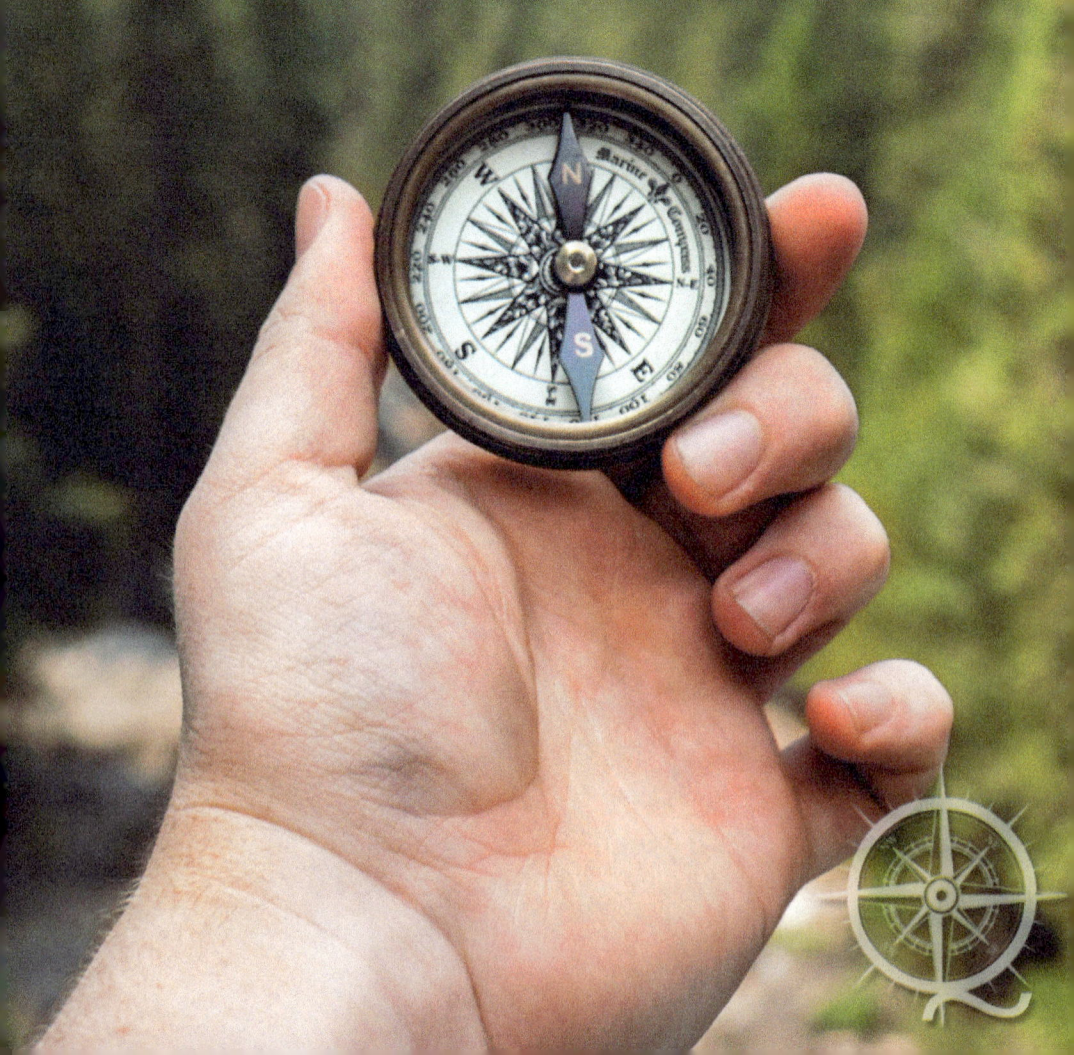

Supplemental

Additional Help on Your Quest to Peace of Mind

Your Anxiety Quest also prepares you for growth in skills and processes needed for sustained peace of mind, reduced suffering, and to help you become your best self. You can be proud of yourself for recruiting help, learning skills, and packing tools for a healthy quest to overcome anxiety.

As a Boy Scout, every month we went on a campout to learn skills for achieving a higher rank and merit badges we needed to become an Eagle Scout, prepared for life and leadership. In my backpack going to Scout camp were all the many things I planned to help me learn, have fun, and be prepared for the constantly changing weather in Missouri. The Scoutmaster had additional supplies just in case the Troop ran out of items necessary for a healthy weekend.

The resource materials below can be viewed as your guide leader handing out references and items you may want to put in your "backpack" of resources for a healthy future.

Table of Contents: Supplemental

References	**121**
Appendix A	**128**
Types of Anxiety (Detailed)	**128**
Generalized Anxiety Disorder	128
Obsessive-Compulsive Disorder	129
Panic Disorder	131
Post-Traumatic Stress Disorder	133
Social Anxiety Disorder	136
Separation Anxiety Disorder	138
Appendix B	**142**
Science of the Brain (Detailed)	**142**
The Limbic System	142
Appendix C	**148**
Assessments for Anxiety (Detailed)	**148**
Generalized Anxiety Disorder: GAD	149
Obsessive-Compulsive Disorder: OCD	150
& Post-Traumatic Stress Disorder: PTSD	150
Social Anxiety Disorder:	153
Separation Anxiety Disorder:	153
Assessing Phobias:	**154**

References

- 21st Century King James Bible. (1994). *The holy bible: The 21st-Century King James version: Containing the old testament and the new testament.* 21st Century King James Bible Publishers.
- ABWE Editorial Staff. (2020, February 19). *47 bible verses about helping others: 7 scriptural themes for generosity.* ABWE. https://www.abwe.org/blog/47-bible-verses-about-helping-others-7-scriptural- themes-generosity
- Adams, C. (2018, January 24). *32 verses to fight fear and anxiety.* One Well Momma. https://wellnessele-vation.com/2018/01/24/32-bibles-verses-for-fear-and-anxiety/
- American Psychological Association. (2017, April). *PTSD assessment instruments.* https://www.apa.org. https://www.apa.org/ptsd-guideline/assessment
- Ankrom, S. (2008, July 6). *The difference between fear and anxiety.* Verywell Mind; Verywellmind. https://www.verywellmind.com/fear-and-anxiety-differences-and-similarities-2584399
- Anthony, K. (2017). *What is EFT tapping? 5-Step technique for anxiety relief.* Healthline. https://www.healthline.com/health/eft-tapping#treatment
- Anxiety Canada. (n.d.). *Self help - cognitive-behavioural therapy (CBT).* Anxiety Canada. https://www.anxietycanada.com/articles/self-help-cognitive-behavioural-therapy-cbt/
- Anxiety Hotline. (2016). PsychGuides.com. https://www.psychguides.com/guides/anxiety-hotline/
- Anxiety hotline number. (2016). Mentalhelp.net. https://www.mentalhelp.net/anxiety/hotline/ Bailey, R. (2018, March 28). *The limbic system and our emotions.* ThoughtCo. https://www.thoughtco.com/limbic-system-anatomy-373200
- Battistin, J. (2016). *5,4,3,2,1 method to reduce anxiety.* Hope Therapy Center. https://www.hope-therapy-center.com/single-post/2016/04/06/54321-method-to-reduce-anxiety
- Caraballo, S. (2019, September 8). *16 bibles verses about courage that'll get you through anything.* Woman'sDay. https://www.womansday.com/life/

- inspirational-stories/g28785488/bibles-verses-about- courage/?slide=16
- Cherry, K. (2021, February 17). *How to forgive yourself.* Verywell Mind. https://www.verywellmind.-com/how-to-forgive-yourself-4583819
- *Diagnosis.* (n.d.). Obsessive-Compulsive and Related Disorders. https://med.stanford.edu/ocd/about/diagnosis.html
- Gordon, S. (2021). *How to live a life of courage.* Verywell Mind. https://www.verywellmind.com/7-ways-to-feel-more-courageous-5089058
- Guy-Evans, O. (2021, April 22). *Limbic system: Definition, parts, functions, and location | simply psychology.*
    - Simplypsychology.org. https://www.simplypsychology.org/limbic-system.html
- Hatala, L. (2018, August 21). *Want to build your emotional courage? Feel into your discomfort.* Women in Leadership for Life. https://womeninleadershipforlife.ca/want-to-build-your-emotional-courage-feel-into-your-discomfort/
- Heshmat, S. (2018). *Anxiety vs. fear.* Www.psychologytoday.com. https://www.psychologytoday.com/ ca/blog/science-choice/201812/anxiety-vs-fear
- Hornthal, E. (2019). *Mindfulness is good, but bodyfulness is better: Here are 3 easy ways to practice bodyfulness.* 30Seconds Health. https://30seconds.com/health/tip/18092/Mindfulness-Is-Good-But-Body-fulness-Is-Better-Here-Are-3-Easy-Ways-to-Practice-Bodyfulness
- Jenkins, S. (n.d.). *How to relax your pelvic floor.* National Association for Continence. Retrieved December 31, 2021, from https://www.nafc.org/bhealth-blog/how-to-relax-your-pelvic-floor
- Krajniak, M. I., Anderson, K., & Eisen, A. R. (2016). Separation Anxiety. In *Encyclopedia of Mental Health* (2nd ed., pp. 128–132). https://doi.org/10.1016/b978-0-12-397045-9.00251-2
- *Limbic system.* (n.d.). Physiopedia. https://www.physio-pedia.com/Limbic_System
- Menéndez-Aller, Á., Postigo, Á., Montes-Álvarez, P., González-Primo, F. J., & García-Cueto, E. (2020). Humor as a protective factor against anxiety and depression. *International Journal of Clinicaland Health Psychology, 20*(1), 38–45. https://doi.org/10.1016/j.ijchp.2019.12.002

- Nelson, C. (2018, November 12). *13 celebrities with anxiety disorders.* EverydayHealth.com. https://www.everydayhealth.com/anxiety-pictures/celebrities-with-anxiety-disorders.aspx
- Nicoletta Lanese. (2019, May 9). *Fight or flight: The sympathetic nervous system.* Livescience.com; Live Science. https://www.livescience.com/65446-sympathetic-nervous-system.html
- Pangilinan, J. (2020, August 9). *105 anxiety quotes to keep you calm when you feel stressed out.* Happier Human. https://www.happierhuman.com/anxiety-quotes/
- Pietrangelo, A. (2014). *List of anxiety drugs.* Healthline. https://www.healthline.com/health/anxiety-drugs
- Powell, D. H. (2004). Treating individuals with debilitating performance anxiety: An introduction.
- *Journal of Clinical Psychology, 60*(8), 801–808. https://doi.org/10.1002/jclp.20038
- PsychDB. (2017, July 11). *Specific phobia.* PsychDB. https://www.psychdb.com/anxiety/phobia
- Rohn, J. (2017, April 30). *3 ways to face your fears with courage.* SUCCESS. https://www.success.com/rohn-3-ways-to-face-your-fears-with-courage/
- Smith, M., Robinson, L., & Segal, J. (2019, May 7). *Panic attacks and panic disorder.* HelpGuide.org. https://www.helpguide.org/articles/anxiety/panic-attacks-and-panic-disorders.htm
- Smith, Y. (2017, September 12). *Generalized anxiety disorder comorbidities.* News-Medical.net. https://www.news-medical.net/health/Generalized-Anxiety-Disorder-Comorbidities.aspx
- *Social Phobia Inventory.* (n.d.). Psychology Tools. https://psychology-tools.com/test/spin
- Stinson, A. (2018, June 1). *Box breathing: How to do it, benefits, and tips.* Www.medicalnewstoday.com.https://www.medicalnewstoday.com/articles/321805#the-box-breathing-method
- Substance Abuse and Mental Health Services Administration. (2014). *Exhibit 1.3-4, DSM-5 diagnostic criteria for PTSD.* Nih.gov; Substance Abuse and Mental Health Services Administration (US). https://www.ncbi.nlm.nih.gov/books/NBK207191/box/part1_ch3.box16/
- Substance Abuse and Mental Health Services Administration. (2016a, June). *Table 3.10, panic disorder and agoraphobia criteria changes from DSM-IV to*

- *DSM-5*. Nih.gov; Substance Abuse and Mental Health Services Administration (US). https://www.ncbi.nlm.nih.gov/books/NBK519704/table/ch3.t10/
- Substance Abuse and Mental Health Services Administration. (2016b, June). *Table 3.13, DSM-IV to DSM-5 obsessive-compulsive disorder comparison.* Nih.gov; Substance Abuse and Mental Health Services Administration (US). https://www.ncbi.nlm.nih.gov/books/NBK519704/table/ch3.t13/
- Substance Abuse and Mental Health Services Administration. (2016c, June). *Table 3.15, DSM-IV to DSM-5 generalized anxiety disorder comparison.* Nih.gov; Substance Abuse and Mental Health Services Administration (US). https://www.ncbi.nlm.nih.gov/books/NBK519704/table/ch3.t15/
- Substance Abuse and Mental Health Services Administration. (2016d, June). *Table 15, DSM-IV to DSM-5 separation anxiety disorder comparison.* Nih.gov; Substance Abuse and Mental Health Services Administration (US). https://www.ncbi.nlm.nih.gov/books/NBK519712/table/ch3.t11/
- Substance Abuse and Mental Health Services Administration. (2016e, June). *Table 16, DSM-IV to DSM-5 social phobia/social anxiety disorder comparison.* Nih.gov; Substance Abuse and Mental Health Services Administration (US). https://www.ncbi.nlm.nih.gov/books/NBK519712/table/ch3.t12/
- The Recovery Village. (2019a, July 1). *Anxiety statistics* (M. Hull, Ed.). The Recovery Village. https://www.therecoveryvillage.com/mental-health/anxiety/related/anxiety-disorder-statistics/
- The Recovery Village. (2019b, September 11). *Anxiety triggers.* The Recovery Village. https://www.therecoveryvillage.com/mental-health/anxiety/related/anxiety-triggers/
- The Recovery Village. (2019c, November 1). *Screening for anxiety disorders* (R. Alston, Ed.). The Recovery Village Drug and Alcohol Rehab. https://www.therecoveryvillage.com/mental-health/anxiety/related/anxiety-screening-tools/
- The Recovery Village. (2020). *10 self-help tips for managing anxiety.* The Recovery Village Drug and Alcohol Rehab. https://www.therecoveryvillage.com/mental-health/anxiety/related/self-help-for-anxiety/Vann, M. (2018, January 11). *How to end an anxiety or panic attack.* EverydayHealth.com. https://www.everydayhealth.com/pictures/how-to-end-an-anxiety-attack/

- Waxenbaum, J. A., Reddy, V., & Varacallo, M. (2021). *Anatomy, autonomic nervous system*. PubMed; Stat- Pearls Publishing. https://www.ncbi.nlm.nih.gov/books/NBK539845/#article-32322.s2
- Wignall, N. (2020, March 16). *How to stop a panic attack before it begins*. Medium. https://medium.com/mind-cafe/how-to-stop-a-panic-attack-before-it-begins-ef46a88da268
- Wright Acupuncture Clinic. (n.d.). *Relaxation and sleep acupressure points*. Wright Acupuncture. Retrieved December 31, 2021, from https://www.wrightacupuncture.co.uk/relaxation-acupressure-points/

LEFT OPEN FOR NOTES

Appendix A

Types of Anxiety (Detailed)

Generalized Anxiety Disorder

Generalized anxiety disorder, otherwise known as GAD, is colloquially known by most laypeople simply as severe, unrelenting anxiety. Affecting about 2.7% of individuals worldwide, over 650 million people are afflicted with GAD (The Recovery Village, 2019a). The symptoms of this disorder are rather straightforward in nature and can be characterized as the usual symptoms experienced by everyone who has anxiety, just to a far more debilitating degree. GAD typically develops from long-term untreated anxiety, which can worsen over time without proper intervention. This type of anxiety is often classified by the presence and severity of these symptoms:

- You have exaggerated feelings of anxiety and worry usually more often than not, over the course of a minimum six month period, about a variety of different events and activities
- These feelings you experience are very onerous, if not impossible, to control
- These feelings are accompanied more often than not, over the course of a minimum six month period, with at least three of the following six physical symptoms:
    - Restlessness or being on edge
    - Irritability
    - Easily fatigued
    - Difficulty with concentration or "mind going blank"

        - Muscle tension
        - Sleep problems
- These feelings and physical symptoms impede and or impair important areas of functioningin your life to a debilitating or clinical degree
- These feelings can not be explained or attributed to another disorder, medical condition, orphysiological effects of a substance

Obsessive-Compulsive Disorder

Nestled comfortably within the family of anxiety disorders, obsessive-compulsive disorder, also known as OCD, is a very interesting yet peculiar type of anxiety. It is one of the least commonly diagnosed disorders, having a prevalence rate of only 1.2% of the population (The Recovery Village, 2019a). This is primarily because OCD is far less easily generalized and the additional manifestations accompanying are highly specific and unique. In fact, it has even been argued by some this disorder is deserving of its own class of disorders, due to the stark differences between OCD and other kinds of anxiety. Despite this discrepancy, for the sake of your understanding, I have opted to include OCD in this section due to its somewhat close proximity symptomatically with other anxiety disorders. Without further ado, OCD typically presents itself as follows:

- You experience the presence of obsessions, compulsions, or both:
    - Obsessions are defined under two dimensions:
        - You experience recurring and persistent thoughts, urges, or images experienced at some point during the disturbance, which is unwanted or intrusivein nature, and result in

you feeling notable levels of distress or anxiety
- You try your hardest to ignore, suppress, or neutralize these obsessions withsome thought or action
  - Compulsions are defined under two dimensions:
    - You engage in repetitive behaviors or mental acts in which you feel heavily inclined to perform by an obsession or rigid rule to be followed
    - These behaviors or mental acts are followed with the idea of preventing or minimizing distress, or even some unwanted event/situation. Also, these behaviors or mental acts have no realistic or tangible connection to what the individual is trying to prevent or minimize and are excessive
- These obsessions or compulsions can take up more than one hour per day and or significantly impede and or impair your ability to function in important areas
- These symptoms can not be explained or attributed to another disorder, medical condition,or physiological effects of a substance

Panic Disorder

Before delving into the details of panic disorder, there are a few things to be clarified about this type of anxiety. First, panic disorder is a blanket term for two disorders called panic disorder and agoraphobia, which can both be distinctly categorized. Whereas just panic disorder is characterized generally by unexpected and recurrent panic attacks, agoraphobia goes one step further to identify specific environmental situations and circumstances triggering panic attacks in some people. In addition to this, panic disorder stems from untreated GAD, meaning you will not just develop panic disorder in a vacuum, but rather as the final stage of severe, untreated anxiety. Because of this, among many other reasons, the prevalence rate of PD is believed to be around 2.7% (The RecoveryVillage, 2019a).

In my experience, almost all of my patients who have had a panic attack fear anotherone so they avoid the person, place, or thing associated with the last one. Finally, in part of explaining the indicators of this type of anxiety, I will also define a panic attack, as well as the common accompanying symptoms. To cover all the bases of this disorder, the criteria of panicdisorder and agoraphobia are both listed here:

- A panic attack can be defined as a sudden rush of powerful discomfort or fear peaking within minutes of initial onset, and at least four, if not more, of these physical manifestations:
    - Chills or hot sensations
    - Trembling or shaking
    - Shortness of breath or feeling of being smothered
    - Sweating
    - Accelerated heart rate, palpitations, or pounding heart
    - Nausea or abdominal discomfort
    - Derealization or depersonalization
    - Chest pain or tightness
    - Fear of dying
    - Feeling of choking

- Numbness or tingling sensation
- Fear of losing control of yourself
- Dizziness, lightheadedness, feeling faint, or unsteadiness
- Panic disorder is classified by you experiencing:
    - Frequent and unexpected panic attacks
    - More than one panic attack has been experienced over the course of one month or one/both of the following:
        - You have a persistent concern about future attacks or their consequences
        - You experience marked maladjusted behavior in concordance with the at-tacks
    - The feelings experienced result in significant imposition and or impairment of important functioning
    - The panic attacks can not be explained or attributed to another disorder, medicalcondition, or physiological effects of a substance
- Agoraphobia, on the other hand, is classified by you experiencing:
    - A noteworthy fear or anxiety about two or more of the following:
        - Standing in line or being in a crowd
        - Being outside the home alone
        - Being in open spaces
        - Using public transportation
        - Being in enclosed spaces, such as shops
    - You actively avoid these situations or circumstances at all costs
        - If you are forced to endure these situations or circumstances, it is done withapparent anxiety or distress over fears of nowhere to escape in the event of experiencing a panic attack and may need a companion to accompany
    - These situations and circumstances almost always invoke anxiety or fear in you

- The feelings of danger experienced by you when faced with these situations and circumstances are grossly disproportionate to the actual threat level presented
- The feelings experienced and avoidant behavior have persisted for at least six months, if not longer, and results in significant imposition and or impairment of important functioning
- The symptoms experienced can not be explained or attributed to another disorder, medical condition, or physiological effects of a substance

Post-Traumatic Stress Disorder

Similar to OCD, post-traumatic stress disorder is characterized by highly specific symptoms. Among the many unique aspects of this disorder, a defining characteristic is the fact to acquire PTSD, someone must experience a marked and intensely traumatic event at some point in their life. Despite PTSD having a sizable list of criteria to be met in order to be professionally diagnosed, it has a prevalence rate as high as 3.6% of the world's population (The Recovery Village, 2019a).

During my career, I have treated many soldiers and first responders who suffer from PTSD, usually as a result of one or more traumatic events. Some of the most intense cases I have treated are firefighters or EMTs who have had to face a situation with a child who is the same age as one of their own children. In addition to firefighters and EMTs, police officers and veterans who have been shot at, seen their friends killed, or wounded commonly are plagued with sleep issues from their PTSD, often re- fusing to go to sleep in an attempt to prevent their horrific, recurring nightmares about their past experiences. The markers of PTSD, in accordance with what has been mostly agreed upon amongst mental health professionals, are:

- You have been exposed to both threatened or actual death, grave injury, or violence in atleast one of the following ways:
    - Exposure through direct experience
    - Exposure through in-person witness, as it occurred to another individual
    - Exposure through being informed the traumatic event was experienced by a closefriend or family member
    - Exposure through incessant or acute in-person experiences with perverse details of the traumatic event, such as first responders addressing fatal accidents
- You have at least one of the following intrusive symptoms associated with the agonizingmemory and only became apparent after the event:
    - Reflexive, frequent, and distressing memories of the agonizing memory
    - Frequent distressing dreams featuring content or similar situations to the memory
    - Dissociative reactions, also known as flashbacks, where you feel and act as thoughyou are re-experiencing the harrowing memory again
    - Psychological and physiological distress is profound and long-lasting when exposed to internal or external cues representing or simulating any part of the memory-related to your affliction
- You maintain a steadfast avoidance of any stimulus associated with the disturbing event, asdisplayed by at least one of the following:
    - Avoidance of any associations, both direct and indirect, including thoughts, feelings,or memories, about the disturbing event

- ○ Avoidance of external reminders stirring these unwanted thoughts, feelings, or memories
- You experience negative changes in ideas and moods associated with the upsetting memory, either beginning or worsening after the upsetting events took place, as evidenced by experiencing at least two of the following symptoms:
  - ○ Inability to recall important details of the memory
  - ○ Consistent and unrealistic negative distortions about yourself and everyone else in the world
  - ○ Distorted interpretations or ideas about the consequences or cause of the traumatic event with you blaming yourself or others
  - ○ Consistent negative emotional state
  - ○ Notable withdrawal or lack of interest in once-loved activities
  - ○ Feelings of alienation or disillusion from relationships
  - ○ Incessant inability to feel positive emotions
- You experience considerable changes in response and awareness associated with the terrifying memory, beginning or worsening after the terrifying event was experienced, as characterized by you experiencing at least two of the following:
  - ○ Contentious behavior with unprovoked bursts of anger is usually expressed in the form of aggression towards objects or other individuals
  - ○ Reckless and or self-destructive behavior
  - ○ Excessive startle response
  - ○ Problems with hyper-vigilance and concentration
  - ○ Problems with sleep
- The duration of the symptoms and criteria listed above have been experienced for a minimum of one month and results in significant imposition and or impairment of important functioning
- The symptoms experienced can not be explained or attributed to another disorder, medical condition, or physiological effects of a substance

Social Anxiety Disorder

Social anxiety disorder, which is sometimes referred to as social phobia, is the most commonly diagnosed form of clinical anxiety. SAD has a prevalence rate as high as a whopping 7.1% across the population, meaning social anxiety disorder affects approximately just over 1.7 billion people worldwide (The Recovery Village, 2019a). This fact should not come as a serious surprise, as it is likely the average person if they thought hard enough, would probably be able to produce an instance, if notseveral, where they experienced a form of social anxiety or social phobia. However, what distinguishes instances of feeling social anxiety versus having social anxiety disorder entirely comes downto the frequency and severity of the indicators experienced by the person. I have found over the years many of my patients are nervous in crowds, in large stores, or in situations like concerts where they believe if something went wrong, they would be helpless or completely out of control. When working with my patients to overcome this, often I ask them to begin with the end in mind, similar to how they will feel going home from an uncomfortable place happy once they have faced it, felt it, and courageously participated in something worth it. To be officially diagnosed with social anxiety disorder, there are a few cues you could pick up on:

- You have feelings of intense anxiety or fear over at least one social circumstance or situation in which you are exposed to the potential criticism of others, which can vary anywhere frombeing observed to social interaction
- These social circumstances or situations often, if not always, invoke feelings of intense fearor anxiety in you
- These feelings of fear and anxiety are wildly disproportionate to the threat beingposed in the social situation or circumstance
- Said social circumstances or situations are ardently avoided by you, otherwise to be forcefullyendured with sharp fear, anxiety, and or distress

- The duration of the symptoms and avoidance listed above have been experienced by you fora minimum of six months and has resulted in significant imposition and or impairment of important functioning
- The symptoms and avoidance experienced by you can not be explained or attributed to another disorder, medical condition, or physiological effects of a substance

Separation Anxiety Disorder

When hearing the term "separation anxiety", the first example coming to the minds of many, would be a child who is overly attached to their parent or a new puppy who cries every time its owner is not in the room with them. While these are both valid examples, having separation anxiety and separation anxiety disorder are two very different things. Separation anxiety disorder, unlike just regular separation anxiety, sits at a prevalence rate of approximately 1.9%, making it almost as common as other anxiety disorders such as GAD and panic disorder (Krajniak et al., 2016). Like with social anxiety, most of us can probably recall a time or two when we experienced separation anxiety from someone or something, but these sporadic experiences alone are nowhere near enough to warrant a clinical diagnosis. Also, separation anxiety, in opposition with what is widely believed, can be experienced by anyone and does not discriminate against age, sex, or gender. For example, I once workedwith a young female patient who refused to go to school, sleep in her own bedroom, or even feel safe out of sight of her mother.

Over time, I found what worked best for her was brief distractions or exposure to short moments alone to be what gave her the most confidence. When small children play Peekaboo, they lack object constancy, which means if they cannot see the other person, the children presume they are alone until they move their hands from their eyes. Similar to my patients, both you and I need the self-confidence we can handle to overcome anxiety. The bench-markers andmanifestations necessary for a person to be officially diagnosed are as follows:

- You experience a developmentally inadequate and inordinate level of anxiety or fear regarding separation from which or whom you are attached, as evidenced by at least three of the following:

- Periodic and exaggerated distress when expecting or experiencing separation from home or figures of attachment
- Periodic and exaggerated anguish over losing figures of attachment or having them come into harm's way
- Periodic and exaggerated anguish over experiencing a disturbing event or circumstance results in separation from figures of attachment
- Insistent apprehension or outright refusal to go out or leave home due to fear of separation from figures of attachment
- Periodic and exaggerated apprehension about or fear of being alone or without figures of attachment at home or in other situations
- Insistent apprehension or outright refusal to go to sleep or sleep away from home without the figures of attachment being close by
- Frequent nightmares involving separation from the figure of attachment
- Frequent complaints of physical symptoms when threatened or faced with being separated from figures of attachment

- The duration of the symptoms and avoidance listed above have been experienced by you for a minimum of six months and has resulted in significant imposition and or impairment of important functioning
- The markers and avoidance experienced by you can not be explained or attributed to another disorder, medical condition, or physiological effects of a substance

LEFT OPEN FOR NOTES

Appendix B

Science of the Brain (Detailed)

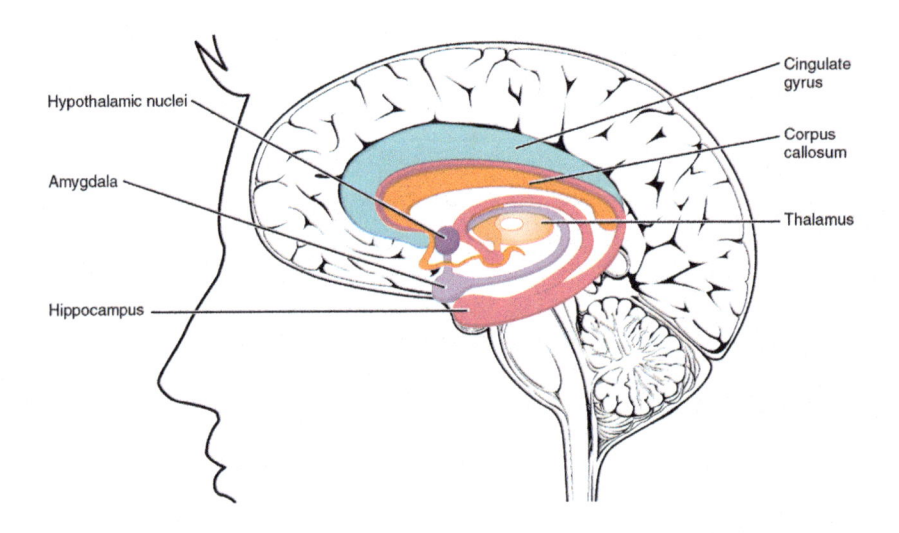

Image Source Credit:
Author: OpenStax College
https://commons.wikimedia.org/wiki/File:1511_The_Limbic_Lobe.jpg
No changes have been made to this image except sizing.
This image file is licensed under the Creative Commons Attribution 3.0 Unported license.

The Limbic System

Buried deep within the center of the cerebrum, which is otherwise known as the collection of the frontal, temporal, parietal, and occipital lobes of the brain, the limbic system is located. Amongst the many functions of this system, it is well known to be a key component of the body's stress response. This is primarily because all the components of the limbic system serve to provide specific functions in and of themselves. These components that make up the limbic system are also speculated to be what creates the bridge between the limbic system and its role with the autonomic nervous system.

The autonomic nervous system, which is also sometimes called the sympathetic nervous system, is the mechanism in your brain responsible for activating a feeling called "fight or flight". When activated, usually in response to threatening stimuli, a series of involuntary physiological processes are engaged in the body. This includes increased blood pressure, heart rate, breathing rate, as well as dilated pupils, and increased perspiration, with marked suppression of digestion, urination, and immunity. All of these functions are engaged with the specific purpose of allowing you to react more quickly or more readily by allowing for greater levels of oxygen to reach your brain in a time of detected crisis.

Aside from stress response, the limbic system is believed to mediate learning, emotionaland behavioral responses, consolidation of knowledge, and forming and storing memories. In my personal experience, all of the years of working with my patients have convinced me when the back of our brains respond to stress by releasing adrenaline and cortisol, they also release some sort of chemical freezing the body and fogging the brain. This chemical has such a strong effect, that it completely clouds the front of your brain and hinders its ability to problem solve in a time of need.

When looking at media, we can easily identify the calm, cool, and collected characters many are so heavily drawn to. Similar to other cool-tempered characters we may see on TV, we can easily see that Batman never loses his cool and always uses his available tools to get himself out of the kinds of situations where you might have feelings of fight, flight, freezing, or fogginess. However, the good thing is, like Batman, you too can learn how to always keep your cool and use your available tools when in a time of crisis!

Moving onto the structure, the limbic system is made up of six substructures: the hippocampus, theamygdala, the cingulate gyrus, the thalamus, the hypothalamus, and the basal ganglia. As stated above, each substructure has its own highly specific function in the limbic system. The one point of controversy about the limbic system is not every professional in the psychology and neuroscience disciplines agrees on whether the thalamus should or should not be included. For the sake of full understanding, information about the role of the thalamus is included in this section, to ensure you have a clear-cut understanding of all the structures playing a role when your limbic system is at work.

The hippocampus has been studied and is believed to serve as the memory center of the brain. Located below all the other substructures of the limbic system, this seahorse-shaped structure plays an essential role in forming and consolidating new memories, as well as recalling ones already stored.

This structure works with feelings of anxiety in a very fascinating way. It is believed the hippocampus is responsible for storing the memories of the trauma or triggers eliciting symptoms of anxiety in response. This, unfortunately, is the reason why many people are unable to completely escape from the stimuli provoking their anxiety—it has been coded into their long-term memory, in which recall can be as intense or unpleasant as actually experiencing the stimulus again. This factor especially affects those of us who are afflicted with PTSD, as the hippocampus plays a vital role in making them relive traumatic experiences through what is known as episodic memories.

Next, the amygdala is another structure within the limbic system. Working closely with the hippocampus in your brain, the almond-shaped amygdala sits next to, but slightly above the hippocampus and is largely responsible for emotion-laden responses including fear, happiness, sadness, anger, and anxiety. Essentially every time you feel an emotion in response to a stimulus, your amygdala is at work. When not mediating regular emotions, the amygdala also acts as the structure that detects and alerts the brain of potential threats and helps to initiate an autonomic nervous system or "fight or flight" response. In the context of how the amygdala interacts with anxiety, this too is a complex process. The amygdala, as it is responsible for emotions, plays a significant role in the consolidation of memories laced with marked emotion. In fact, the strength of the level of emotional arousal at the time of a person experiencing an event has a direct influence on the retention of the memory inthe future.

If you are experiencing intense emotions or distress during a certain situation or circumstances, you are more likely to vividly remember what took place when asked to recall. On top of this, it has become increasingly apparent to researchers that the amygdala has a much larger affinity for consolidating negative memories over positive ones, and it can make associations between avoidance and fearful stimuli after very little repetition. As time passes and more negative memories are consolidated, however, the amygdala changes to become unable to adequately detect actual threats versus whatis a perceived one, which results in feelings and symptoms of anxiety. It is believed the work put in by the amygdala and the hippocampus together makes up the majority of how PTSD works.

The role of the thalamus in the limbic system is a small but important one. The thalamus serves as ahub of connections for many different substructures of the limbic system to the brainstem to otherentirely unrelated mechanisms in the brain. Almost all signals sent from one structure to another arerelayed through the thalamus on the way. Aside from acting as a connection hub, the thalamus is involved in the regulation of motor responses and sensory perception, as one of the many processing centers for these two mechanisms. The hypothalamus, on the other hand, plays a much bigger role in the function of the limbic system. Located right below the thalamus, the most basic function of the hypothalamus is to maintain a balanced internal state.

The hypothalamus is responsible for many automatic processes within the body including thirst, arousal, hunger, blood pressure, heart rate, and body temperature. In a time of distress, signals from the hypothalamus send the autonomic nervous system into action. In addition to this, the hypothalamus mediates a great deal of the hormones produced by the endocrine system. Since this tiny structure is responsible for a multitude of bodily functions, it is known as an information integration center that considers and is responsive to, a wide array of different types of stimuli. As a result, the hypothalamus is a highly sensitive structure and can easily misinterpret stimuli and signals when you are under high stress or in distress. In the context of anxiety, the overactive response of the hypothalamus, which results in feeling anxiety, can predominantly be attributed to the inaccurate signals being detected and transmitted by the hippocampus and amygdala.

Somewhat akin to the role of the thalamus, the cingulate gyrus is an integral structure of the limbic system and provides connections between current stimuli and previous memories and emotions. Rather than detecting emotions or consolidating memories, the cingulate gyrus works to create accurate predictions as to when aversive stimuli will be faced via monitoring bodily responses to all stimuli. While an amygdala usually becomes more sensitive with more exposure to negative stimuli or experiences, the cingulate gyrus will execute how you actually respond to the stimulus or situations.

This structure can become less or more sensitive over time and therefore can result in inappropriate responses to certain situations such as failing to have a fearful response in dangerous situations. In the case of anxiety, the cingulate gyrus works hand in hand with all of the other limbic system sub-structures to produce disproportionate responses and therefore anxious symptoms when triggered.

The final structure of the limbic system covered in this section is the basal ganglia. Instead of being just one structure, it is a group of several substructures that primarily function to mediate voluntary movements, balance, and posture. Made up of structures called the nucleus accumbens, the ventral tegmental area, and the ventral pallidum. The basal ganglia is also believed to play roles in regulating some aspects of emotional and cognitive behavior, as well as rewards and reinforcements. Because of this, it is believed this multi-structured system is a fundamental player in habit formation.

This belief is what helps with explaining exactly what the basal ganglia contribute in terms of its role in feeling anxiety. The basal ganglia helps with priming your brain for repetition and even has a preference for repetitive behavior, whether repetition is intended or not. As a result, each time the limbic system inadequately detects aversive stimuli and inappropriately reacts to said stimulus, the chances of the same thing happening again are increased. This means virtually every single time you experience an anxious response, you are actually priming your brain for it to happen again in the future.

As you can see, the limbic system plays a very crucial role in anxious responses. Through a developed understanding of how this system works to create anxious symptoms, however, you now have the knowledge necessary to begin learning how to effectively counteract the processes of specific substructures and greatly minimize or even eradicate anxious responses across many circumstances and situations.

Appendix C

Assessments for Anxiety (Detailed)

Compared to just fifty years ago, today there are endless amounts of assessments available. These range from self-assessment questionnaires online to formal in-person conversational assessments with a mental health professional. As more and more research is produced to work toward understanding anxiety, more and more hyper-specific assessments seek to targetspecific kinds of anxiety can be created. This progress has allowed both researchers and people withanxiety to develop a more sound understanding of how anxiety works and what the most effective intervention promotes life-long relief.

One of the most commonly used forms of assessment in examining anxiety disorders is by matching patient symptoms to criteria listed in a textbook called the DSM-5. Also known as the fifth edition of the Diagnostic and Statistical Manual of Mental Disorders, this textbook is the official guide published by the American Psychiatric Association and is widely regarded as containing the officially accepted criteria for the diagnosis of mental illness. Much of the tools and assessments used by professionals today are based on the content presented in the DSM-5, as a means of ensuring uniformity across the field of psychology in testing and diagnosis.

Before jumping right into assessments specified for certain anxiety disorders, there are two tests to be considered, which can help quite significantly if you feel a little unsure of where to begin in starting your assessments. First and foremost, before pursuing specific anxiety disorder assessments, it is best to establish you are truly afflicted with anxiety and are not being misconstrued with another mental illness.

To establish this, the Beck Anxiety Inventory (BAI) is especially helpful. One of the key attributes of this twenty-one-item self-report questionnaire is questions are worded in a manner allowing for a clear distinction to be made between an individual who is suffering from anxiety versusan individual who is suffering from depression. Should you take this assessment and find you are in fact within the anxious category rather than the depressive one, the next recommended assessment to consider pursuing is the Hamilton Anxiety Rating Scale (HARS).

The Hamilton Anxiety Rating Scale is a fourteen-item self-report questionnaire created to be an assessment not exclusive to GAD and can measure the severity of general anxiety, whether diagnosed or not. Completing the HARS will give you a better idea of which kind of assessment would be best suited for you to pursue, should you further believe you have a specific anxiety disorder. These assessments can be found online free of charge and can help significantly with clarifying your anxiety. This can be especially helpful in the circumstance your scores are above the normal range and can reinforce your desire to seek out a professional guide on your journey to recovery.

Generalized Anxiety Disorder: GAD

When looking to assess if you may have generalized anxiety disorder, there are a considerable number of tests to choose from, but some are far more popular than others. An example of a popular assessment is the Generalized Anxiety Disorder Scale (GAD-7), which is a seven-item self-report questionnaire with questions surrounding the frequency of anxiety symptoms and behaviors. In addition to the GAD-7, there is also another similar six-item self-report questionnaire called the Generalized Anxiety Disorder Severity Scale (GADSS).

The only difference between the Generalized Anxiety Disorder Scale and the Generalized Anxiety Disorder Severity Scale is the latter includes questions about the severity of symptoms as well as questions about the frequency. Although theseassessments are officially geared towards examining GAD, they can also be easily applied to assess-ing related kinds of anxiety such as panic disorder, due to the close nature of symptoms if you are afflicted with either.

Obsessive-Compulsive Disorder: OCD & Post-Traumatic Stress Disorder: PTSD

For officially recognized afflictions such as OCD or PTSD, there are far fewer accurate assessments in circulation due to the specific criteria for diagnosis. For OCD, an assessment largely viewed as thegold standard for obtaining accurate information on the severity of symptoms is the Yale-Brown Obsessive-Compulsive Scale (Y-BOCS). The Y-BOCS test is a ten-item clinician-administered questionnaire with questions about several dimensions of obsessions and compulsions. Rather than actually being a test of diagnosis, the Y-BOCS test has the purpose to provide greater insight or information helpful in determining a diagnosis. Regarding screening for PTSD, there is a handful of both self-report assessments and clinician-administered assessments.

For self-report assessments of PTSD, there is the Davidson Trauma Scale (DTS) which is a seven-teen-item questionnaire for the frequency and severity of the symptoms experienced. In addition tothis, a more recently developed self-report assessment growing in popularity of use is the PTSD Checklist for DSM-5 (PCL-5), which is a twenty-item questionnaire assessing the core symptoms usually experienced by those with PTSD. On top of this, the PCL-5 can be used to monitor changesin symptoms before, during, and after treatment.

In terms of clinician-administered assessments for PTSD, there are two of particular interest due totheir pervasiveness and proximity to the diagnosis criteria expressed in the DSM-5, which are the Clinician-Administered PTSD Scale for DSM-5 (CAPS-5) and the PTSD

Symptom Scale Interview (PSS-I-5). The CAPS-5 assessment is currently the most popular clinician-administered assessment used to diagnose PTSD and is made up of thirty items posed to help the clinician develop a deeper understanding of your symptoms and feelings.

The PSS-I-5 in contrast is a much simpler assessment of seventeen items on reviewing someone's history of trauma in the hope of being able to isolate the single traumatic event named responsible for the distress the person is facing at a point in time. I personally regularly use these for the evaluation of anxiety disorders and often find my patients are usually not aware of the frequency, intensity, duration, and impact on their lives of PTSD and anxiety.

For example, if we look up at the black night sky and see all those little white dots, we call them stars. An astronomer sees patterns like the big dipper, Orion, and Aquarius. Similarly, when I show a patient the "constellation" of their symptoms that defines a disorder, then treatment can be personalized and more effective.

Anecdotes: 1/27/2022

OCD

One form of obsession is addiction and the compulsive behavior used to lessen anxiety. I worked with a couple who owned a business and budgeted $10,000 per month to gamble at a casino. They rationalized their compulsions because they received "comps" of show tickets, hotel nights, spa treatments, dinners, and an occasional cruise. My perception was to cut out the middle man and spend their hard-earned money on their entertainment. Their argument was if they went to a concert or movie, they could not win any money.

Finally, they did the math and felt foolish for the time and money wasted at the casino. To see the difference between what little they won and the value of what they were comped from their losses, they bottomed out and started recovery. They went through some psychological withdrawal at first, not getting to see their "friends" (the employees they got to know by being frequent flyers at the games). After they trespassed themselves, they were hurt no one at the casino contacted them or showed any further interest in them, which helped them reinforce their decision to quit going.

PTSD

A combat veteran from the wars in the Middle East had been terrified during the beginning of an attack. Between two buildings, a latrine had been set up for the soldiers. They took turns with other guys who watched out for them when they could literally be caught with their pants down. He had undressed and felt exposed and vulnerable when a rocket exploded very close to them, without any warning, leaving him helpless to defend himself or others. He did not get injured physically by the battle, but he avoided going to the bathroom to prevent the traumatic event from terrifying him again.

When he returned home, he had nightmares and flashbacks, which he tried to avoid by not sleeping or using a restroom. His turning point from suffering his post-traumatic stress was an attitude of gratitude centered on his friends and him not getting wounded or killed by those rockets. He wept about feeling selfish about his fears instead of focusing on the miracle none of them were hit. His mission was to keep his prayers and orientation on his fellow service members, their families, and those less fortunate. His payoff was he finally felt relieved.

Social Anxiety Disorder:

In the case of assessing and measuring social anxiety disorder, there also exists a handful of tests. The most well-known assessment commonly used to evaluate both social anxiety disorder and performance anxiety is called the Liebowitz Social Anxiety Scale (LSAS), which is a twenty-four-item self-report questionnaire divided into two subscales, with one scale posing questions about performance anxiety and the other about situational social anxiety. In addition to the LSAS, there is also the Social Phobia Inventory (SPIN), which is a simple self-report seventeen-item questionnaire to establish the severity of the feelings and symptoms experienced by the person.

Separation Anxiety Disorder:

While years of research have successfully yielded several accurate assessments to measure social anxiety disorder, the same unfortunately cannot be said for separation anxiety disorder. More often than not, a combination of assessments that look at both generalized anxiety disorder and social anxiety disorder to assess separation anxiety disorder, as it is believed to be the disorder overlapping with the two. However, this is not to say assessments specifically for separation anxiety disorder do not exist, but rather the existing ones are not adequate enough to cover symptoms of separation anxiety regardless of age and are typically more geared towards assessing children. Interestingly, most people afflicted with separation anxiety are contagious, meaning others around them are affected by what they say and do. Often we think of children hiding behind their mothers' skirts.

Another form of separation anxiety has an impact on kindergarten teachers, who complain about young mothers on the first day of school who exhibit a lot of separation anxiety about "cutting off the apron strings" and trusting the school with their baby. Sometimes this even happens again 18 years later, when the student heads off to college and the empty nest fosters anxiety for mothers who have a change in their role.

Assessing Phobias:

When looking to assess specific phobias, three main self-report assessments are utilized. Both the Phobia Questionnaire (PHQ), which is fifteen items, and the Fear Questionnaire (FQ), which is twenty-four items, aim to assess the degree of someone's avoidance of a certain object or situation out of fear or distress. The Specific Phobia Questionnaire (SPQ), on the other hand, is an alternative option to the PHQ and FQ; which is a forty-five-item assessment to measure the severity of fear levels experienced across many different situations and objects.

Although it may not be the nicest thing to do, sometimes people cannot help but compare how their phobias are exhibited personally to

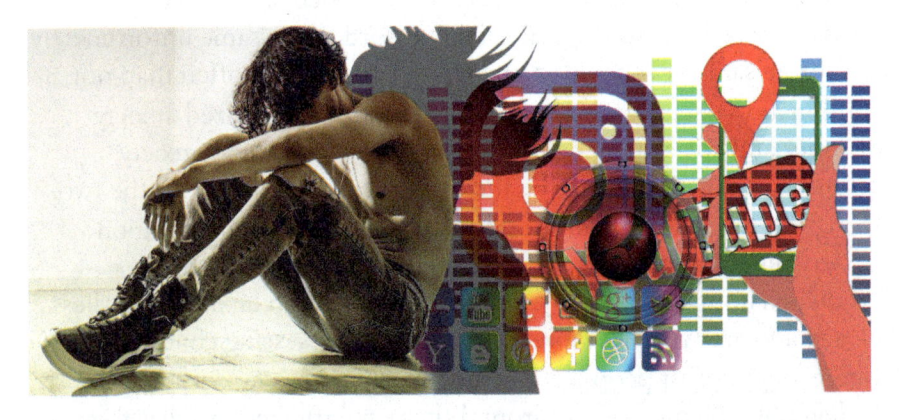

Image Source Credit:
Author: Geralt
https://pixabay.com/photos/social-media-social-network-3762538/
No changes have been made to this image except sizing.
This image file is licensed under the Pixabay license.

how they are exhibited in the media by actors. An example of this would be thinking something like, "at least I am not as bad off as Jack Nicholson in 'As Good As It Gets." Aside from comparison, simply just looking at the common or novel phobias, can be a personal point of interest.

Over 400 distinct phobias are recognized and there are new ones I come across in my line of work regularly, such as nomophobia, which is the fear of not having your cell phone with you. Sadly, there have been teenagers in Spokane who have been grounded from their phones and committed suicide—maybe they see it as a sixth finger getting amputated. We have compassion for anyone so fearful of missing out they would prefer death, but when we look at the social media and texts, death does not seem warranted for the content they felt they could not live without.

LEFT OPEN FOR NOTES

Made in the USA
Columbia, SC
07 July 2023